The Office Effect

Handbook

EASY SOLUTIONS FOR WORK-RELATED PAIN

By Craig Zuckerman & Matt Williamson

ISBN: 1456479245
ISBN-13: 9781456479244

This book is intended to provide helpful information and motivation to our readers, and is a reference guide only. This book is not meant to be used as a medical manual, nor should it be used to diagnose or treat any medical condition. For diagnosis or treatment of any medical problem that you know or suspect you have, consult a physician. Additionally, the information provided in this book is not intended to be a substitute for any treatment, including but not limited to any exercise routine and/or dietary regimen that may have been prescribed to you by a doctor. All forms of exercise present some inherent risks. The authors, editors, contributor and publisher of this book are not responsible for any specific health needs that may require medical supervision and are not liable for any damages or negative consequences from any treatment, action, application, or preparation by or to any person reading or following the information and exercises in this book. Several exercises in this book require the use of a *red band*, a length of flexible surgical rubber that provides even, adjustable resistance. Check your red band before each exercise for any defects, tears, or cuts that can cause the band to snap, which may result in an injury. It is important not to take risks beyond your level of experience, aptitude, training, and fitness. References are provided for informational purposes only and do not constitute endorsement of any websites or other sources.

Any and all web addresses and phone numbers provided in this book were accurate at the time this book was finalized for printing.

Printed in the United States of America
CreateSpace

Contributor - Charles Schiavone
Method and Exercise System Developer - Craig Zuckerman

Exercise & Office Photographs - Peter Dokus
Cartoons & Illustrations - Sasha Dix
Book Cover and Interior Design - Matt Williamson, CreateSpace

Acknowledgments

I would like to thank my wife, Lori, for putting up with me and the long hours while writing this book. If it wasn't for her, Matt, Charlie, and I would never have gotten together to create this project. It is her support that keeps me sane, her love that keeps me warm, and her positivity that keeps me smiling. I want to thank Paige and Don for their love and amazing input that helped make this project the best it could be. To Jeremy and Hila, without their support and guidance, I would not have been able to make this project work. I must thank all of my clients for listening to me babble about *The Office Effect* all year long and for being honest with their thoughts and patient with my schedule; they are all my inspiration. To Chyrel, for encouraging me to head down this path, even though I wasn't always the most receptive apprentice. And to my parents, who have always supported me through every adventure, who have always loved me no matter what I chose to do, and who have been there for me through all my trials and tribulations. Last but not least, to Matt and Charlie, my partners at CMC Fitness Solutions, thank you for helping me to put what's in my head on paper and create this project.

Craig Zuckerman

I would like to thank Lisa for her support during this process. I know it wasn't easy. To Jay, Tanya, Pierre, Brooke, and all my other clients who listened with care and offered valuable advice, I thank you. A special thanks to my attorneys, Michael and Rockell, for their wisdom, generosity and guidance throughout this project. Of course, I have to give massive amounts of credit to my mom, who has been my rock from day one, literally. Finally, I need to thank my partners at CMC Fitness Solutions for their dedication and ability to take a joke. Thanks fellas.

Matt Williamson

First and foremost, I would like to thank my wife, Meighan, for her incredible support, understanding and helpful input during the countless days and nights I worked with my partners, Craig and Matt, on this book. Needless to say, my contributions to this book and the build-out of our company wouldn't have been possible without her. Additionally, I would like to thank my dad, Joe, for all of his mentoring throughout my career, which greatly influenced and tuned my skill sets, allowing me to achieve publishing this book and launching our company. I would also like to thank our family and friends who read drafts of our book and provided us with useful feedback that helped shape this book. Especially my mother-in-law Michelle, my sister Trish, my brother Frank, Craig's wife Lori, and Craig's clients and friends Don and Paige. Finally, my thank you wouldn't be complete without thanking Craig and Matt. I continue to be impressed with their work ethic, knowledge, and enthusiasm. I couldn't have asked for better partners.

Charles Schiavone

About the Authors

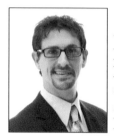 **Craig Zuckerman** has been working in the rehabilitation and personal training world for over a decade. He originally studied Dance and Kinesiology at Missouri State University where he received a BFA in Theatre and Specialized Minor in Dance. After incurring a knee injury and having subsequent knee surgery, Craig worked closely with the Midwest Sports Medicine Clinic's doctors and Physical Therapists to create a program for MSU's dance department, keeping dancers in optimal shape and health.

Two years later, Craig received a full Stott Pilates Certification in all levels and apparatuses. After moving to Los Angeles, Craig became the director of a Pilates-based rehabilitation center, Rapid Rehab International. There he created a program specifically for spinal disorders while working with doctors from the Spine Institute in Santa Monica California and the Spine Center at Cedars-Sinai.

Using biomechanical analysis and kinesiology, he constructs programs specific to his client's injuries. Within these programs, he has created hundreds of specialized exercises that combine Pilates, cardio, weights, and stability apparatuses to form unique and challenging workouts. Craig gives master classes and lectures across the nation about various subjects, like his specialized hybrid Pilates and rehabilitation techniques. Not only has Craig helped rehabilitate people with M.S., Parkinson's, hip and knee replacements, and spinal disorders, he has also trained corporate executives, Olympic athletes, professional golfers, dancers, and celebrities.

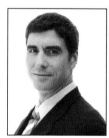 **Matt Williamson** is a National Academy of Sports Medicine Certified Personal Trainer and Corrective Exercise Specialist. He has been a fitness professional for over ten years and has changed the lives of many of his clients. Matt's knowledge of the human body comes not only from his education in the world of fitness, but also from his education and experience in the entertainment industry. He has a BFA in Theatre and Dance from Missouri State (where he met Craig) and an MFA in Acting from UCLA. He has appeared on numerous television shows, movies, and even on Broadway.

Matt also developed a keen awareness of biomechanics through ten years of martial arts training in Jeet Kune Do. Matt has taught kickboxing, boot camps, and group classes, and has logged thousands of hours of private training. His clients have included billionaires, celebrities, children, cerebral palsy patients, soccer moms, grandparents, and war veterans. He has worked with Michael Thurmond (*Six Week Body Makeover* as seen on TV) and trained several of the participants on the ABC series *Extreme Makeover*.

Contents

The Office Effect

Part IV: Fix It for Life! *The Office Effect Exercises*

Part V: Fix It Outside the Office

If you work like this,

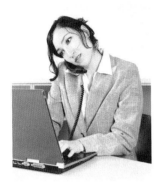 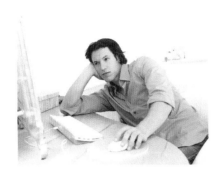 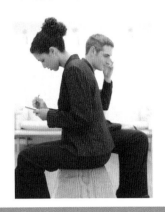

and you feel like this,

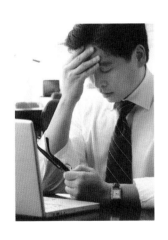 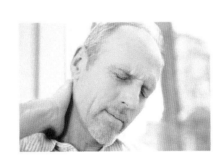 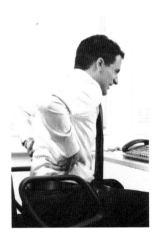

then you are feeling...

The Office Effect

What is The Office Effect?

The Office Effect is the negative impact of work-related repetitive stress on the body. It's the bad posture, aching joints, headaches, and fatigue that come from sitting at a desk all day. It affects how you feel, look, and perform. In other words, *the daily grind is grinding you down.*

Why should I fix it?

The man pictured is only thirty-five years old and has postural Kyphosis, the medical term for a hunched back. This disorder is caused by muscular imbalances due to repetitive stress, such as poor posture. Although this disorder is becoming more prevalent every day, it can be avoided, if you have some awareness and basic knowledge. That is what this book is for.

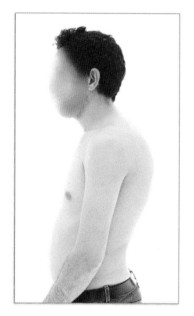

Kyphosis

Symptoms of *The Office Effect*:

Kyphosis	Loss of Bladder Control
Lordosis	Loss of Bowel Control
Edema	Osteoarthritis
Sciatica	Straight Spine Syndrome
Muscle Spasms	Spondylolisthesis
Subluxation	Thoracic Outlet Syndrome
Radiculopathy	Carpel Tunnel Syndrome
Fascia Build-up	Patella Femoral Syndrome
Herniations	Degenerative Disc Disease

These may seem extreme, but they are all possible and indicative of the impact that repetitive stress can have on your body.

Our solution!

We decided that *The Office Effect* was important enough to tackle as an international health issue, on par with obesity and smoking. CMC Fitness Solutions is dedicated to bringing an awareness of the problem to the working world, along with a comprehensive system for feeling, finding, and fixing *The Office Effect*. With more and more people becoming dependent on computers and PDAs, including children, we can no longer afford to ignore what our lifestyle is doing to our bodies. The good news is that although the problem is severe and widespread, the solution is relatively simple. A few minor adjustments and some simple exercises can help relieve and even prevent *The Office Effect*.

Part I
Common Causes of
The Office Effect

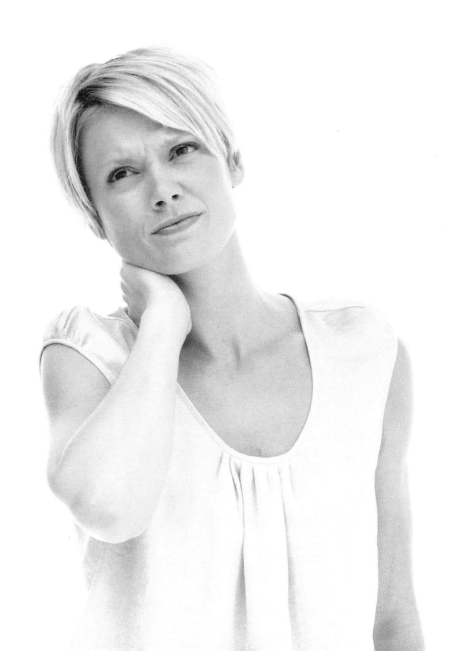

True Stories of *The Office Effect*

Client Story #1: The Case of the Crossed Leg

I had a client who came to me with sciatic pain running down her right leg. When I asked her what her daily routine was, she said she spends about six-plus hours a day in front of her computer for work, and that's usually when the pain started to kick in.

I knew that Sciatica is commonly caused by the piriformis muscle in the buttocks spasming. So I asked if she happened to sit at her desk with her right leg crossed often. She thought for a second and then replied, "Yes, I do. In fact, I always cross my right leg. How did you know?" I then replied, "I'm psychic!" I, of course, was kidding.

The piriformis muscle rotates the leg outward, but when you sit with your legs crossed for long periods of time, the muscle gets put into a stretched position, weakening it and destabilizing the pelvis. Often times, the piriformis then seizes up or spasms which in turn causes it to pinch down on the sciatic nerve, causing Sciatica. So I had my client stop crossing her legs and showed her some simple exercises to strengthen the muscles around her hips, pelvis, and lower back, including the piriformis. After two weeks, all her pain had gone.

Now, if any of her symptoms flair up, like after a long day at her computer where she may not be so conscious of her posture, she takes a break, does *The Office Effect 10 Minute Exercise Program* and her pain goes away. She even showed her husband some of the exercises when he had back pain, after working in the yard, and he got some pain relief too!

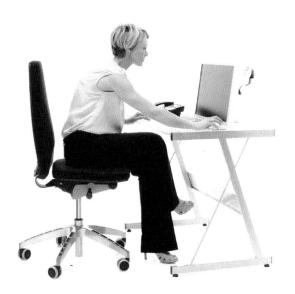

> *"When I do the exercises they get me out of pain. When I'm more consistent with them, they keep me out of pain and it only takes me five to ten minutes to do them. You just have to do it."*
>
> *Kathy,*
> *Client*

Repetitive stress is the silent enemy that is with us at work, at home, and all points in between. It can be a position or posture that is held for too long, such as slouching at your desk or using your PDA. It can also be a movement that is performed over and over, such as twisting in your chair many times a day, or turning your head hundreds of times while transcribing. You may have a headache, backache, sore shoulder, or any number of other conditions and never realize that they stem from a simple repetitive stress at work or at home. You're in pain and you don't *really* know why!

Improper Postures

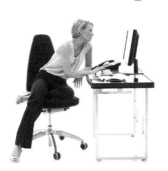 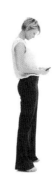

Repetitive Movements

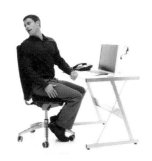 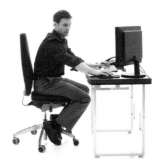

Repetitive stress exists in almost every aspect of our lives. Unfortunately, most people can't even identify a single repetitive stress in their workplace, let alone in their daily lives. They just keep going through the same routine day after day without considering the long-term consequences. If you let repetitive stresses chip away at your health, don't be surprised when your doctor gives you bad news. But it doesn't have to be that way.

You can avoid future problems by taking action now. The first indication of The Office Effect is pain...

Pain

Pain is the body's way of telling you that something is wrong.

Pain caused by *The Office Effect* usually occurs when a nerve is impinged or "pinched." When this happens, the nerve sends a signal through the spine to the brain in the form of pain. Unlike touching a hot surface, we usually don't immediately react to this type of pain. If we did, we would all have perfect posture and alignment.

As we ignore it, the nerve becomes distressed and the next sensation we feel is a tingling (this is common in the fingers after too many hours of typing). As time goes on, the tingling turns to numbness as the nerve loses its ability to relay information efficiently. Finally, all communication through that nerve gets cut off, resulting in loss of muscle control. We call this, "The Pain Progression."

The Pain Progression

PAIN ⇒ TINGLING ⇒ NUMBNESS ⇒ LOSS OF MUSCLE CONTROL

Imagine not being able to lift your coffee cup!

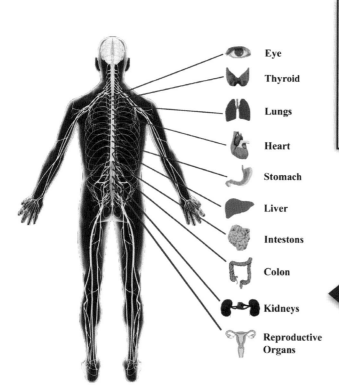

Eye
Thyroid
Lungs
Heart
Stomach
Liver
Intestons
Colon
Kidneys
Reproductive Organs

Unfortunately, most of the time, we ignore the pain and/or take a pill to make it go away. This doesn't solve the problem; it merely masks it.

Remember...

The nervous system connects to every major system in the body. So if a pinched nerve in your neck makes your finger tingle, a pinched nerve in your back could release your bowels. Just ask the corporate executive with the spastic colon.

Most of the pain associated with *The Office Effect* comes from pinched nerves. But how does a nerve get pinched in the first place? It happens when too much pressure is put on the nerve by the surrounding tissue. Here are the most common nerve pinching scenarios.

Muscle Spasm (Knots)

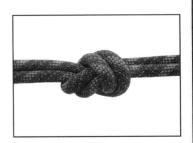

Muscle spasms are involuntary contractions of the muscle, which can last minutes, hours, or days. There are many causes of muscle spasms, such as disease, dehydration, and excessive exercise, but we are more concerned with spasms caused by weakened, stressed, or over-worked muscles. When these spasms occur, they put excess pressure on the nerves, causing pain.

Disc Herniation

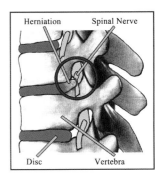

Disc herniations are bulges in the soft tissue between the vertebrae. The discs provide flexibility for the spine and act as shock absorbers. When the spine is placed in an improper position, as is the case with poor posture, the excess pressure can force the disc to bulge, pinching nearby nerves as they exit the spine, causing pain.

Fascia

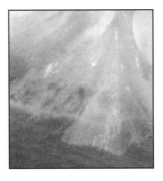

Fascia is a web-like tissue that naturally forms in our body. It is the translucent film that surrounds muscles and helps them retain their shape. However, if a muscle is forced to hold a position for extended periods of time, the body will overproduce fascia, which thickens and hardens like concrete. The body does this because it is the easiest way to hold that position. Unfortunately, the hard fascia will pinch nerves and lock the muscle in place making movement difficult.

Posture

Posture affects how you look and feel, as well as how others perceive you. Bad posture compresses your organs and spine, destabilizes your joints, and causes pain—not to mention that it just looks bad. It's an energy black hole that caves in on itself, sending a message to everyone you meet that you are stressed, self-conscious, tired, or even unhealthy.

> *"If you could make yourself taller, more attractive, more approachable, and happier without pills, surgery, or therapy... why wouldn't you?"*
>
> *Jay,*
> *Client*

Same person...different messages.

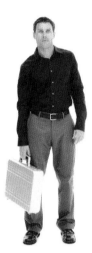

✓ Tired
✓ Stressed
✓ Self-conscious
✓ Possibly Sick
✓ Over-worked
✓ Unapproachable

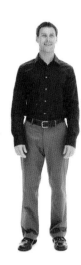

✓ Attractive
✓ Confident
✓ Knowledgeable
✓ Well Rested
✓ In Control
✓ Go-getter

Some Common Improper Postures

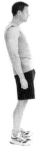

Swayback

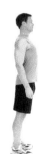

Military

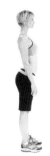

Lordosis

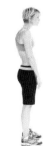

Kyphosis

Look in the mirror or ask your doctor to help you check for any of these common improper postures. If caught and dealt with soon enough, these conditions can be reversed before they become permanent.

Many of the problems associated with *The Office Effect* start with posture, or more specifically, the impact of posture on the shape and function of the spine. The spine protects the spinal cord, which is the information super highway of the body. It has other important functions as well. It acts as a structural foundation and a shock absorber, kind of like the frame and suspension of a car. If it is forced to change its shape due to repetitive stresses, disease, or developmental disorders, it can no longer perform its duties effectively and efficiently.

How the Spine Works

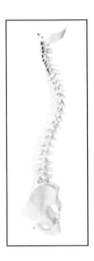

The spine has a natural "S" curve that allows it to dissipate the weight of the body and the external forces that act upon it. This shape allows it to be flexible while maintaining its strength. It is constructed as a series of movable joints divided by fluid filled pillows called discs. These discs are vital to the spine's mobility and ability to absorb shock, but are also the source of most spine related pain. When they are put under continual uneven pressure they can herniate, or bulge out to one side, like squeezing a water balloon. When this occurs, they can put pressure on any one of the many nerves that branch out from the spinal cord, causing pain and forcing the surrounding musculature to tighten up in order to protect that area.

How Does *The Office Effect* Change the Spine?

The Office Effect changes the shape of the spine by forcing it to hold incorrect positions for extended periods of time. If you thrust your head forward daily in order to see your monitor better, eventually it will stay there, changing the shape of the cervical spine (neck). If your keyboard is too far away, forcing you to hunch your upper back, it will change the shape of your thoracic spine (mid/upper back). If you spend hours rounding your lower back, you guessed it, it will change the shape of your lumbar spine (lower back). With time, this incorrect shape will be held by the formation of hardened fascia tissue in the surrounding muscles, making it difficult and painful to reverse. It can also lead to disc degeneration and changes in the vertebrae themselves (which are irreversible).

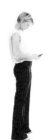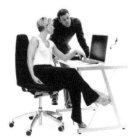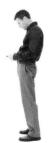

Musculoskeletal Disorders (MSDs)
According to California Occupational Safety & Health Administration...
- Work-related MSDs are the leading cause of lost-workday injuries and compensation costs in the country.
- MSDs account for 34 percent of all lost-workday injuries and illnesses.
- More than 620,000 lost-workday MSDs are reported each year.
- MSDs account for $1 of every $3 spent for workers' compensation.
- MSDs each year account for more than $15 to $20 billion in workers' compensation costs. Total costs add up to as much as $60 billion.

Sitting
According to the American Cancer Society...
Sitting for long periods of time raises your risk of dying regardless of your level of physical activity. Research found over a fourteen-year study that women who sit for six hours a day were 37 percent more likely to die during the length of the study than women sitting for three hours a day, and 18 percent more likely for men. Study author Alpa Patel, Ph.D., says that these harmful effects of sitting can be prevented by simply getting up and moving every hour.

Cancer
According to the American Cancer Society...
Regardless of your age being active is an important part of staying healthy. It may also lower your risk for certain types of cancer. With that, they suggest the following to help you become and stay active:
- It's as important for kids to be active as it is for adults. Kids develop habits early in life, and you can help give them a healthy start.
- Regular physical activity is easier to fit in than you may realize and can significantly lower your lifetime risk for cancer—and heart disease and diabetes, too.
- No matter when you start, *exercise improves health*. Even people who start exercising later in life appear to gain many of the same health benefits as people who have exercised their whole lives.

Pain and Depression
According to the Mayo Clinic...
Pain and the problems it causes can wear you down over time, and may begin to affect your mood. Chronic pain causes a number of problems that can lead to depression, such as trouble sleeping and stress. Disabling pain can cause low self-esteem due to work, legal, or financial issues. Depression doesn't just occur with pain resulting from an injury. It's also common in people who have pain linked to a health condition such as diabetes or migraines.

Part II
Solutions

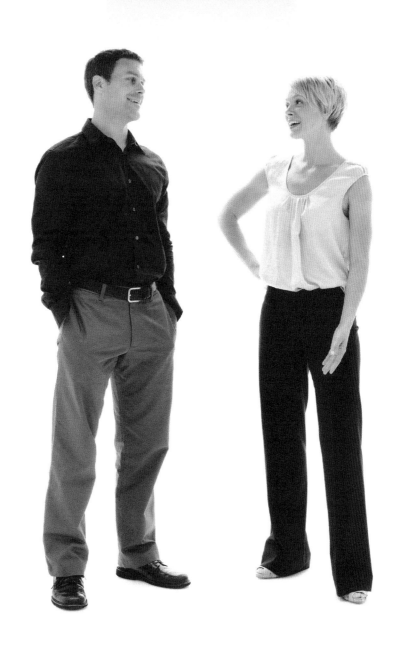

Feel It, Find It, Fix It

The *3 F's* is a method that we developed over many years of research and development for easily identifying pain, identifying the cause of pain, and taking the necessary steps to relieve pain and correct improper posture. This system makes it easy to take control of your body and your environment and stop the pain progression.

Feel It

What is my body telling me?

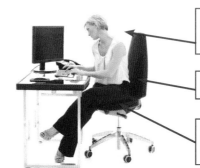

Right side neck pain and shoulder pain

Lower back pain

Left side pain shooting down her leg (Sciatica)

Find It

What is causing my pain?

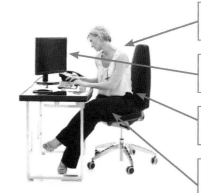

Rotated head and hunched shoulders

Computer screen on right side

Lower back rounded

Left leg always crossed over

Fix It

How can I relieve pain and improve my posture?

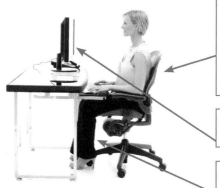

Correct posture: Get lower back to curve properly with exercise and an ergonomic chair or lower back support

Move computer screen directly in front

Uncross legs

Feel It

What is my body telling me?

Your body is trying to tell you that something is wrong!

Acknowledge and identify your pain or tension. Start at the top of your head and work your way down your body. Gently move your head, neck, shoulders, elbows, wrists, hips, knees, ankles, and feet. Be specific, make a note of what movements cause you pain, on what side of the body you are feeling it, and when you feel it the most. Do any of the conditions below feel familiar?

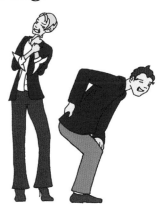

Do you experience any of these aches and pains?

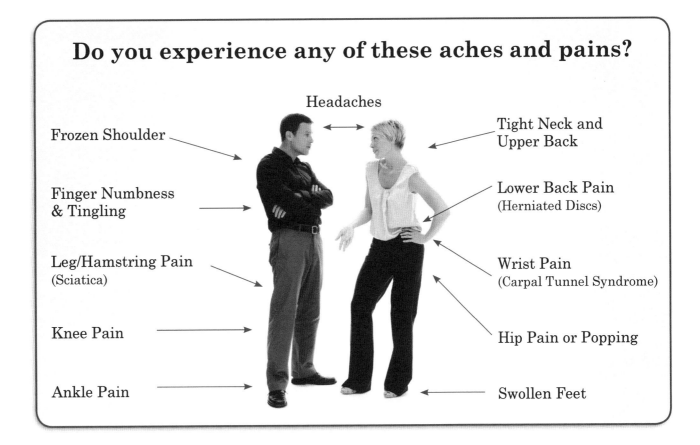

Headaches

Frozen Shoulder

Tight Neck and Upper Back

Finger Numbness & Tingling

Lower Back Pain (Herniated Discs)

Leg/Hamstring Pain (Sciatica)

Wrist Pain (Carpal Tunnel Syndrome)

Knee Pain

Hip Pain or Popping

Ankle Pain

Swollen Feet

Solutions

Find It

What is causing my pain?

Become a detective. The first place to look for clues...your posture.

Do you have a forward head? Hunched shoulders? Rounded low
If you do, it could be the cause of your pain!

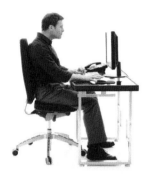 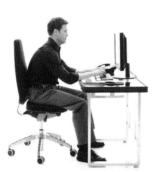 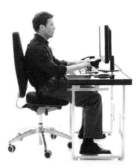 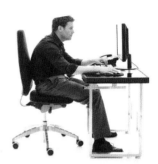

Forward Head   Hunched Shoulders   Rounded Lower Back   All Three

Now that you've taken an honest look at your posture, it's time to figure out what environmental factors may be contributing to the problem. Ask yourself these questions.

1. Is your screen too far away?

2. Is your keyboard/mouse too far away?

3. Do you have proper lower back support?

4. Are your legs tucked under your chair?

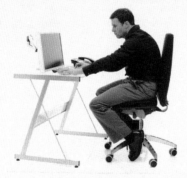

1. This will cause your head to move forward.

2. This will cause your shoulders to roll forward.

3. Without proper lumbar support, the lower back can round.

4. This can limit blood flow, cause edema (swelling), and put pressure on the sciatic nerve.

This is a very important step because it directly addresses the causes of pain and poor posture. Once you become a detective and begin to ask the right questions, you will realize that the aches and pains you feel every day have a simple explanation.

Fix It

How can I relieve pain and improve my posture?

Make simple changes to your environment and daily habits.

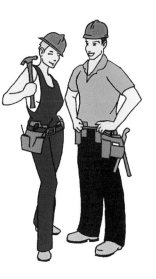

By changing just one repetitive stress and employing the specific exercises we have developed, you can relieve pain and improve your posture.

We know that it is not realistic to expect you to sit at your desk with perfect posture all the time. However, we can give you the tools to return to a proper position whenever you want.

For many people, sitting correctly feels wrong and sitting incorrectly feels right. Stay committed and give it time. Eventually, that situation will reverse itself and you will look, feel, and perform better.

Use the picture below to help you set up your working environment so that it is ergonomically correct. If just one component is off, it can become a painful repetitive stress.

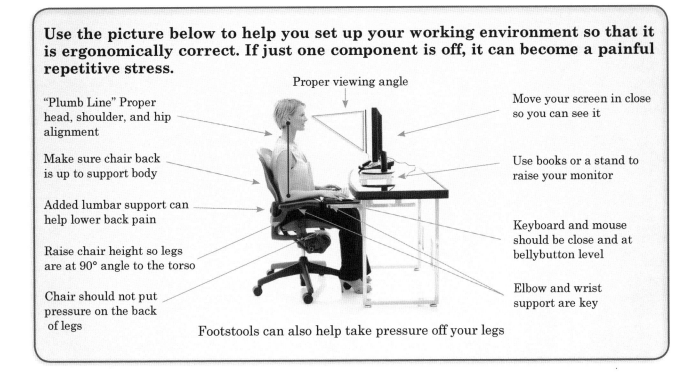

Proper viewing angle

"Plumb Line" Proper head, shoulder, and hip alignment

Make sure chair back is up to support body

Added lumbar support can help lower back pain

Raise chair height so legs are at 90° angle to the torso

Chair should not put pressure on the back of legs

Move your screen in close so you can see it

Use books or a stand to raise your monitor

Keyboard and mouse should be close and at bellybutton level

Elbow and wrist support are key

Footstools can also help take pressure off your legs

Quick Ergonomic Fixes

These are some of the most common desktop ergonomic mistakes that we have seen. *Compare these pictures with your workspace.*

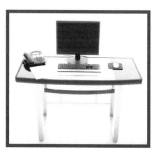

=

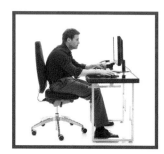

✓ Monitor too far away
✓ Mouse too far away
✓ Keyboard too far away

✓ Forward Head – Neck Pain
✓ Hunched Shoulders – Shoulder Pain
✓ Rounded Back – Back Pain

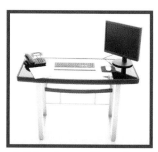

=

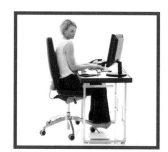

✓ Monitor off to the side
✓ Mouse too far away
✓ Keyboard too far away

✓ Turned Head – Neck Pain
✓ Hunched Shoulders – Shoulder Pain
✓ Rounded Back – Back Pain

See how a few easy changes can begin to relieve pain and improve posture.

Get a headset for your phone

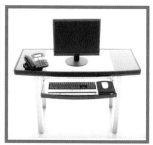

=

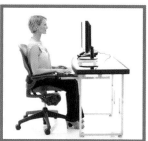

A keyboard tray can put your keyboard and mouse at the right level

✓ Monitor close enough to see clearly
✓ Keyboard and mouse are on a tray, or chair is high enough to bring them close to the body at bellybutton level

✓ Head, neck, shoulders, and elbows are aligned
✓ Weight is evenly distributed
✓ Pain is relieved
✓ Posture improved

With today's insane pace at the office, coupled with how much technology (laptops, broadband/VPN, PDAs, etc.) has us tethered to our jobs, we are literally non-stop. This level of intensity makes it easy to get stuck at your desk for hours on end at the office and even at home. Your metabolism slows, your cholesterol rises, your joints stiffen, and that's just the beginning.

An easy way to combat this is to simply get up and move for a few minutes. Here are a few suggestions.

Wiggle, Bounce, and Roll

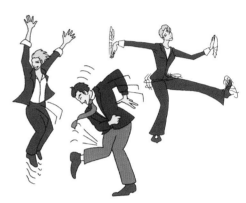

Sounds silly, we know, but it works. Just take a few seconds every couple of hours to stand up, wiggle your whole body, bounce up and down, and roll your joints. It will get the blood flowing, loosen the muscles and joints, and make you feel like a kid again. It's also a great warm-up before exercising! *You'll even burn calories and lower your cholesterol.*

Drink Water

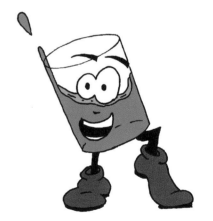

You've heard this a million times; well here's number one million and one. We all know that water is good for us and most of us will admit that we don't drink enough of it. Keep a case of bottled water at your desk. If you don't like the taste, add a lemon slice or even flavored vitamin drops—whatever it takes to get you to drink it. It will keep your muscles from tightening, your joints lubricated, and it will raise your metabolism, helping your body function more efficiently. *About one fluid ounce of water for every two pounds of body weight is your goal!*

Find a Way to Relax

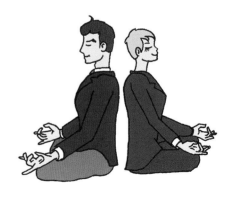

Having the weight of the world on your shoulders is terrible for your posture. Take a deep breath and find some time, even a moment, just to reset—at least once a day. Release your tongue from the roof of your mouth. Go for a walk outside. Listen to some music. Call your spouse or kids, *anything to allow your mind and your body to take a break from the stress of the day.*

The Office Effect Exercises!

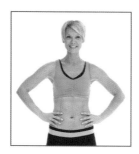

An ergonomically correct work environment is very important but it is not the only step. *Fix It* actually has two parts. Adjusting your workstation may provide immediate relief but in order to *fix it for life* and achieve long-term results, you must strengthen your body.

If your body is not strong and stable enough to maintain proper alignment, you will slip right back into your old ways no matter how ergonomically correct your workstation is.

Just 10 Minutes

Let's be honest, some people love to exercise; some people hate it. No matter how you feel about it, anyone can manage ten minutes. The bottom line is this: exercise will make you feel better both physically and emotionally. Life is too short to go around looking bad and feeling pain if you don't have to. A committed, comprehensive approach will allow you to take control of your body, return to proper posture and alignment, relieve your pain, and elevate your mood and productivity.

You Are an Athlete! Seriously.

No matter how sedentary your job may be, think of yourself as a professional athlete. A pro tennis player trains their body to move fast in many directions, swing a racket with force and efficiency, and maintain their stamina. That's their job. If your job means that you have to sit at a desk for hours on end, focus your attention, and maintain proper posture, then you have to train your body to do that as well.

Exercise = Lifelong Results

In Part III of this book, you will see *The 3 F's Method* in action. After you have identified your pain, identified the cause of your pain, and adjusted your environment, we will always recommend that you perform our exercises to *fix it for life*. In Part IV, you will find *The Office Effect* Upper and Lower Body Exercise Series. These are low-impact exercises that are specifically designed to relieve pain and improve posture for the rest of your life.

Part III
Relieving Pain & Correcting Posture

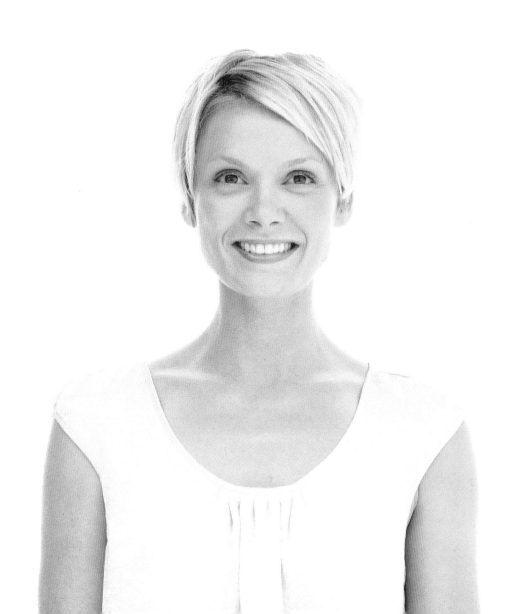

Applying Feel It, Find It, Fix It

The 3 F's Method is an easy step-by-step way to feel, look, and perform at your best. We understand that it is unrealistic to expect you to have perfect posture and maintain correct ergonomics all the time. However, when the aches and pains that result from hours in front of the computer start to slow you down, you will have a way to get back on track.

Use the following section to help locate your pain. Follow the steps, try the suggestions, and develop an awareness of your body and environment. Make a commitment, be consistent, and start relieving your pain and correcting your posture.

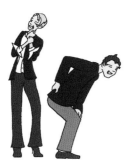 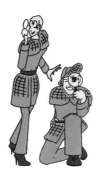 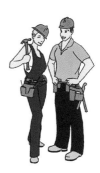

Applying The 3 F's Method

Feel It

This may be the easiest of the *3 F's*, but it is also the most important. It's the beginning, the moment that you decide that you don't want to live in pain anymore. Just by recognizing then identifying what you are feeling everyday, you take the first step toward relief.

Find It

Find It can actually be fun if you let it. You get to become a detective and root out the criminal elements that are causing you pain. We will give you the tools to be an effective detective. You will learn to spot pain inducing repetitive stresses a mile away. And we will show you how posture can affect the way you feel and how others perceive you. *Find It* allows you to learn a lot about yourself and your environment.

Fix It

It's time to do something about pain and poor posture! This section will show you how to make the changes that will stay with you for the rest of your life. The habits that you form will have a significant impact on your body over time. Fix the problem now to avoid bigger problems later. However, to *fix it for life*, you must exercise and strengthen your body to endure a career behind a desk and in front of a computer.

Headaches & Neck Pain

Feel It

✓ **Neck pain**
✓ **Headaches**
✓ **Tingling and/or numbness in the fingers**

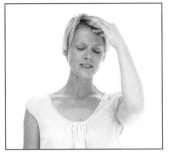
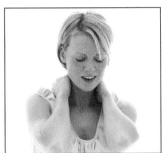

If you experience pain and stiffness in your neck and/or headaches, you are not alone. In addition to neck pain, many people also experience tingling in the fingers. These are the first two steps in *The Pain Progression*.

Find It

✓ Monitor too far away
✓ Forward Head

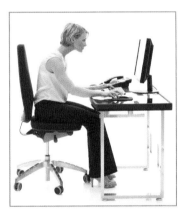

Check your posture.
For every inch that your head is forward from its correct position, it adds an additional ten pounds of weight that your neck has to support. This puts tremendous strain on the neck muscles, causing painful spasms. This can also result in disc herniations that pinch the nerves and can cause tingling. *This neck position can even reduce oxygen intake up to 20 percent.*

Why is your head forward?
The most common cause of Forward Head is improper monitor position. If your monitor is too far away, your head will naturally move forward in order for you to see it better.

Fix It

✓ **Move monitor closer**
✓ **Chin Tucks**

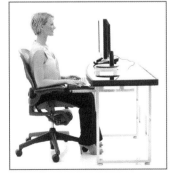
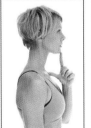
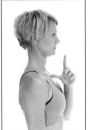

Chin Tucks

Taking the third step is easy.
Move your monitor closer so that you can see it with your head and neck in proper alignment.

Fix It for life!
Integrate Chin Tucks (see *The Office Effect* Upper Body Exercise Series) into your daily routine.

Movement-based Neck Pain

Feel It

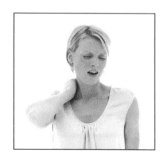

✓ Neck pain, mainly on one side
✓ Neck pain when moving the head
✓ Tingling and/or numbness in the fingers

- Do you feel more pain on one side of your neck?
- Do you feel pain when you turn to one side only?

If you do, you may be experiencing a repetitive movement stress. The more specific you are when identifying and describing your pain, the easier it will be to *Find It* and *Fix It*.

Find It

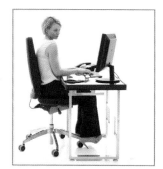

✓ Monitor positioned off to the side
✓ Turning head many times a day while transcribing

One of the most common of these repetitive movements is transcribing. This usually happens one of two ways:

- Is your monitor positioned directly in front of you and the material that you are transcribing off to the side?
- Is your monitor off to the side and the material that you are transcribing from directly in front of you?

Either of these two scenarios can cause you to turn your head to the side hundreds of times a day. Simply having your monitor off to one corner of your desk will cause you to hold your head in a rotated position for long periods of time. When your head is slightly rotated and/or tilted, and you have neck pain or tingling fingers, it could be the result of transcribing or your screen being positioned in the corner of your desk.

Fix It

✓ Move monitor to the center
✓ Switch the side the document holder is on periodically
✓ Split transcribing material with the monitor
✓ Perform *The Office Effect* Upper Body Exercise Series

If you do a lot of transcribing, split the center of your desk with the monitor and document holder so both sides of your neck get equal rotation from right to left. Performing *The Office Effect* Upper Body Exercise Series will trigger the stabilizing muscles of the neck, reducing pain.

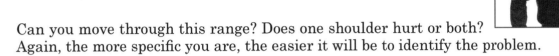

Feel It

✓ **Pain and stiffness in one shoulder**
  • **Gently move shoulders through their basic range of motion.**
  • **Raise both arms in front of you to shoulder height.**
  • **Raise both arms to the side to shoulder height.**

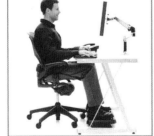

Can you move through this range? Does one shoulder hurt or both? Again, the more specific you are, the easier it will be to identify the problem.

Find It

✓ **Mouse is too far away**
✓ **Raised shoulder**
✓ **Bursitis or Frozen Shoulder Syndrome**

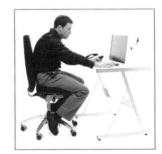

Reaching out for long periods of time with your arm to control your mouse can cause the muscle in your shoulder to spasm from over work and holding a continual contraction. Over time, this can cause Bursitis and Frozen Shoulder Syndrome.

Bursitis is the swelling of a small fluid filled sack that exists in your joints, such as your shoulder and hip. It acts as a cushion, but when continual pressure is applied to the joint from the surrounding muscles being in spasm, the bursa will become inflamed and cause pain.

Frozen Shoulder Syndrome is a painful condition that results from the body over producing fascia in the shoulder. Eventually, this will prevent you from lifting your arm.

Fix It

✓ **Move mouse closer to the body**
✓ **Consider a trackball mouse**
✓ **Perform *The Office Effect* Upper Body Exercise Series**

Move the mouse closer to your body so that your elbow lines up vertically with your shoulder. This will relieve the strain on your "mouse" shoulder. Adjusting your armrests to support your elbow and forearm will also reduce strain. Perform *The Office Effect* Upper Body Exercise Series to strengthen and rehabilitate your shoulder. Consider a trackball mouse to minimize the repetitive movement.

Upper Trap & Shoulder Pain

Feel It

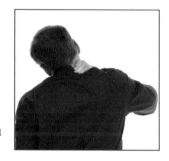

✓ **Pain in upper traps/neck**
✓ **Pain in neck**

The upper trapezius muscle spans from your neck down to your shoulder. Knots or spasms often occur in this muscle, causing pain that radiates into the neck and head. If you've ever felt like you had a softball between your shoulder and neck then that's what we're talking about.

Find It

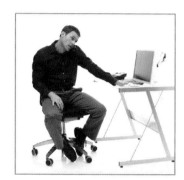

✓ **Keyboard and mouse too far away**
✓ **Chair too low or keyboard to high**
✓ **No armrests**
✓ **Raised shoulders**

- If it looks like you are wearing your shoulders as earrings, or like you play for the Dallas Cowboys, you're probably over working your upper trapezius muscles (traps), which lift your shoulders up.
- If your keyboard or mouse is too far away, you may be continually engaging this muscle as you reach for your keyboard and mouse.
- If your keyboard is too high or your chair is too low, causing your elbows to be lower than your keyboard, you may be constantly engaging your traps in order to lift your shoulders and arms high enough to reach your keyboard.
- One of the most common causes of this type of pain is stress.

Fix It

✓ **Move keyboard and mouse closer**
✓ **Raise chair or use keyboard tray**
✓ **Raise arm rests**
✓ **Perform *The Office Effect* Upper Body Exercise Series**
✓ **Meditate**

Raise your chair or get a keyboard tray so your elbows are in line with your wrist. This position is best obtained when your keyboard is at bellybutton height and your armrests are high enough to support your arms. *The Office Effect* Upper Body Exercise Series can not only help to pull your shoulders down, but simply by exercising, your brain goes into relaxing Alpha waves and your body releases endorphins.

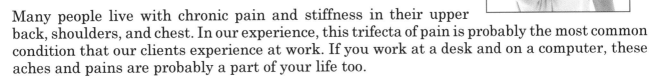
Chest & Upper Back Pain

Feel It

✓ **Pain between shoulder blades**
✓ **Pain in back of shoulder joint**
✓ **Pain in front of shoulders**
✓ **Pain in chest muscles**
✓ **Cold, pale hands**

Many people live with chronic pain and stiffness in their upper back, shoulders, and chest. In our experience, this trifecta of pain is probably the most common condition that our clients experience at work. If you work at a desk and on a computer, these aches and pains are probably a part of your life too.

Find It

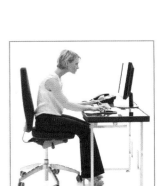

✓ **Keyboard too far away/too high**
✓ **Monitor too low and/or too far away**
✓ **Laptop resting on lap**
✓ **Hunched posture**

Hunching over your desk causes the muscles that run along the spine to work overtime to keep your body from falling forward and crashing into your desk. If held continually, these muscles will spasm, pinching down on the nerves exiting the spine, causing pain. Fascia will eventually start to build up over the upper back muscles, locking them and your spine into a condition known as **Kyphosis.**

Thoracic Outlet Syndrome: Tight chest and neck muscles can put pressure on the nerve and artery that run under your collarbone. This diminishes communication to the brain and limits blood supply to the arm and hand.

Fix It

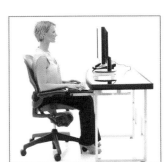

✓ **Move keyboard close to body at bellybutton level**
✓ **Move monitor up to proper level (use stand or books)**
✓ **Perform *The Office Effect* Upper Body Exercise Series**

Your keyboard should be right in front of your bellybutton. Ideally, you should have armrests on your chair that are high enough to support your arms. Use a monitor stand or even a phone book or two to raise your monitor up to eye level. *The Office Effect* Upper Body Exercise Series will help give you the strength and stability to maintain proper posture.

Lower Back Pain

Feel It

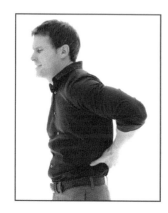

✓ **Pain centralized at lower spine**
✓ **Pain radiating up or out through lower back**
✓ **Pain on one side of lower back/upper hip**

A dull radiating ache, stiffness, and sharp stinging pain are all common lower back pains. Sometimes you may feel a funky pain right on top of one of your hip bones in your lower back. When you touch this area, it will feel like you're bruised. Many times you don't feel these pains until you change positions, like when you stand up from sitting in a chair.

Find It

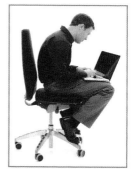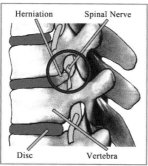

✓ **Rounded lower back**
✓ **Herniated disc in lower back**
✓ **Lifting while twisting**

Rounding your lower back is a sure way to get lower back pain. It puts pressure on the discs in your lower back and can eventually cause them to herniate. The lower back muscles will seize up in an attempt to prevent the herniation from getting worse, giving you radiating lower back pain.

- One of the number one causes of a lower back herniation is bending over to pick something up and twisting as you lift it.
- Weak lower back, abdominal, and hip flexor muscles will allow for a rounded lower back.
- If your chair is too far from your desk or your backrest isn't supporting your lower back, you may be contributing to your bad posture and lower back pain.

Fix It

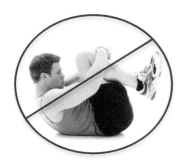

✓ **Lumbar support**
✓ **Lift items straight in front of you**
✓ **Don't stretch your lower back when it hurts**
✓ **Perform *The Office Effect* Lower Body Exercise Series and Press-Ups**

You may feel like stretching your lower back when it hurts, but think twice. Stretching can actually make it worse by allowing a herniated disc to bulge further. Performing *The Office Effect* Lower Body Exercise Series will give your back the strength to support you efficiently.

Hip, Buttocks, & Groin Pain

Feel It

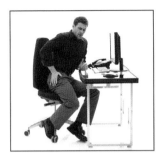

✓ **Pain in front hip crease or inside hip joint**
✓ **Pain in tailbone**
✓ **Pain in top of hip bone, on one side of lower back**
✓ **Pain in groin/bladder region**

If you feel a pain in your buttocks, top of your hip bone in your lower back, the front crease of your hip, or in your groin, you may be having an SI joint instability. The SI joint is where your lower spine (sacrum) meets your pelvic girdle (iliac), hence the term SI joint.

This intersection between the two bones can shift out of place, causing the surrounding muscles of the pelvis to spasm. These muscle spasms will cause pain and tension in multiple areas of the hip, such as the tailbone. This shift can also impinge the nerves that connect to your legs, ankles, and feet, as well as your intestines, colon, and reproductive organs.

Find It

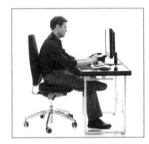

✓ **Crossing one leg**
✓ **Rounding lower back while sitting**
✓ **Sitting on one hip**
✓ **Standing with weight supported on only one leg**

The following can cause SI joint instability:

1. Sitting with the same leg crossed
2. Sitting with a rounded lower back
3. Sitting/standing with your weight shifted onto one hip/leg
4. Sitting with one hip hiked up on the desk

When your SI joint is unstable, you may notice:

1. One hip being higher than the other
2. Your hips may be twisted due to the rotation of the hip bone and spasming muscles
3. One leg may appear to be shorter than the other

Fix It

Lumbar Supports

✓ **Support weight equally while sitting and standing**
✓ **Don't cross same leg for extended period of time**
✓ **Use lumbar support**
✓ **Perform *The Office Effect* Lower Body Exercise Series**

Many fixes for SI joint instability can happen simply by stopping certain repetitive stresses. To *fix it for life*, *The Office Effect* Lower Body Exercise Series should be done in its entirety at least twice a week to stabilize and align the SI joint.

Sciatica

Feel It

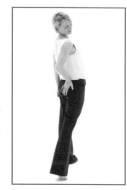

✓ **Pain in buttocks**
✓ **Shooting pain down leg**

Sciatica is usually felt as a sharp pain, deep inside your buttocks, or as a sharp shooting pain down the back or side of your leg. Often it is described as a feeling of hot electricity running down the leg.

Find It

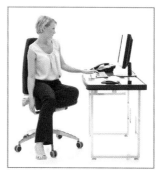

✓ **Crossed legs**
✓ **Spasm in piriformis muscle**
✓ **Rounded lower back**

Sciatica is caused by disc herniations in the lowest two vertebrae of the spine and/or from an impingement on the sciatic nerve. This is usually the result of a spasming piriformis muscle, which is located deep under the buttocks.

- Continually crossing one leg can cause the piriformis muscle to be over stretched. If this happens, it can recoil into spasm and impinge the sciatic nerve that runs under it.
- Sitting with your lower back rounded can also cause pressure on the SI joint, which is where your spine meets your hip bones. This can cause that joint to spread or shift, which, in turn, can cause the piriformis muscle to spasm in an attempt to protect or realign the SI joint. The spasming piriformis will then impinge the sciatic nerve, sending shooting pain down the back of the leg. This is often referred to as **Piriformis Syndrome**.

Fix It

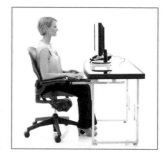

✓ **Don't cross your legs**
✓ **Use lumbar support**
✓ **Perform *The Office Effect* Lower Body Exercise Series**

To fix these conditions, try not to cross your legs. If you must cross your legs, refrain from doing so for long periods of time and switch the leg you're crossing periodically. A lumbar support can help, but you need to make sure you're sitting against it so it can support you. However, the best way to maintain proper posture and prevent Sciatica is to strengthen the muscles that hold your body's posture. *The Office Effect* Lower Body Exercise Series will strengthen the lower back muscles as well as the piriformis muscles, allowing you to relieve sciatic pain.

Carpal Tunnel Syndrome

Feel It

✓ **Pain in the wrist/arm and tingling in the fingertips**

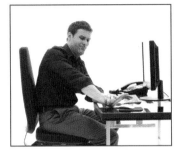

Carpal Tunnel Syndrome is a type of painful nerve damage caused by compressing and irritating the median nerve in the wrist. The nerve is compressed inside the carpal tunnel, a bony canal in the wrist that provides passage for the median nerve to the hand. The irritation of the median nerve is usually due to pressure from the transverse carpal ligament (a band that runs across the underside of the wrist).

Find It

✓ **Arms are unsupported**
✓ **Wrists are bent at an angle**
✓ **Head and shoulders are forward, pinching the median nerve**

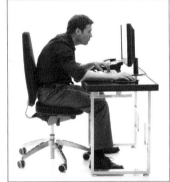

In some cases, the symptoms of C.T.S. (tingling and numbness in the fingers, pain in the wrist and arm) occur because the median nerve is irritated at some point other than the carpel tunnel. This nerve runs from the fingertips, up through the length of the arm, under the clavicle (collarbone), and into the cervical spine. Pinching this nerve can happen anywhere along its route. For example, a forward head can cause the nerve to be pinched in the neck. Chest and shoulder muscles can also spasm, pinch the nerve, and cause similar pain and tingling as Carpal Tunnel Syndrome.

Fix It

✓ **Use armrests**
✓ **Adjust keyboard height to bellybutton level**
✓ **Use wrist supports**
✓ **Perform *The Office Effect* Upper Body Exercise Series and Median Nerve Stretch**

> **Median Nerve Stretch**
>
> - Straighten your arm, pulling it back and away from your torso, fingers spread out, wrist bent back.
> - Tilt your head slightly away from your arm for a more intense stretch.

Make sure that your wrists and elbows are supported. They should not be angled vertically or horizontally. Perform *The Office Effect* Upper Body Exercise Series and consult your doctor if the pain is severe and/or ongoing. *Remember: the idea is to prevent Carpal Tunnel Syndrome, not to treat it.*

"Did you know...just ten minutes of exercise, a few times a week, can give you the pain relief you've been wanting."

Craig Zuckerman

Part IV
Fix It for Life!

The Office Effect Exercises

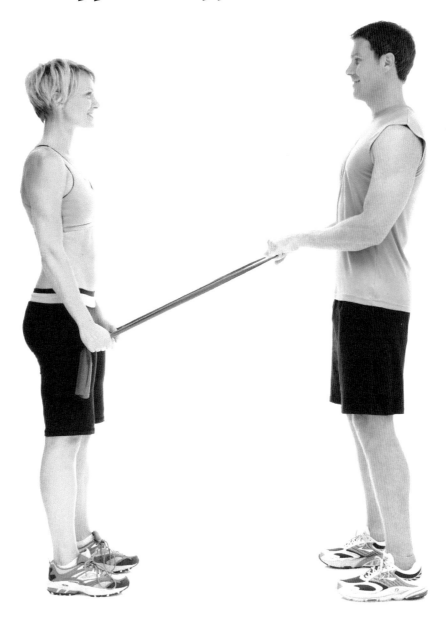

Both of *The Office Effect* Exercise Series are designed to help you get out of pain. They strengthen your stabilizing muscles, allowing you to maintain proper posture throughout your work day. The muscle fibers we target burn fat as their fuel and are exercised in a way that allows them to maintain their functionality over long periods of time.

The Golden Rules of Exercise

PAIN = STOP	If you feel a sharp pain at any time during an exercise...*Stop!*
SLOW AND STEADY	Keep your movements slow, controlled, and in the proper range of motion—no jerking and no popping! *This can hurt your joints.*
BREATHE	Inhale on the preparation, exhale on the exertion. Be sure to breathe as you are moving; don't hold your breath. *Proper oxygen levels prevent fatigue and lactic acid build-up (cramping).*
ENGAGE YOUR ABS	Gently pull your bellybutton in and up on every exercise that you perform. Proper breathing will help with this. *At no time during an exercise should your abs be relaxed.*
FORM IS KEY	Keep your eyes open and use a mirror to make sure that your movement and alignment are correct.
NEVER LOCK YOUR JOINTS	A locked joint can injure easily.

Why our system works!

These exercises are put together in a specific order, incorporating a system we developed, **Counter Muscle Balancing**™. Simply put, when working one muscle or group of muscles of a joint, you should then work the opposing muscle or muscle group of that same joint. This allows all the surrounding muscles of a joint to be worked in tandem, stabilizing the joint and giving your body the balance it needs to get out of pain and prevent further injuries. For example, if you work your abs, you should then work the muscles of your lower back so that one side does not become dominant and create an imbalance. This is the key to our exercise system.

How to Do Our Exercises

Which exercises should I do?

The simple answer...*all of them*. You can just exercise the area that affects you, however, we suggest that you do both the Upper and Lower Body Exercises Series in order. This will help balance your body as a whole. Perform these exercises two to three times a week and it will help you prevent or relieve *The Office Effect* in just ten minutes.

How many repetitions should I do?

We recommend a certain number of repetitions for each exercise. This is a good place to start. If you can do more, feel free, but don't sacrifice form for reps. In most cases, the number of reps will be *between ten and twenty-five*.

How do I know what muscles I'm working?

The muscle charts will show you what areas you are supposed to be working. These are low intensity exercises so you may not feel a "burn" or "pump" associated with more intense exercises such as lifting weights. *You should feel a warm, tight sensation in the highlighted area about half way through each set.* If you don't feel anything in the highlighted area, check your form. Use the muscle chart as a guide to show you where you should be focusing your attention.

The Versatile Red Exercise Band

Several exercises require the use of a red band, a length of flexible surgical rubber that provides even, adjustable resistance. Be sure to check your band before each exercise, as any tears or cuts can cause the band to snap, causing injury. If you find yourself struggling to do the first few reps of an exercise, you may have too much tension on your band. Give it some slack and continue with the exercise. If the exercise is too easy, you may want to add some tension to the band to increase the resistance. Just remember, these exercises are targeting stabilizer muscles, so twenty reps are always better than eight really hard reps.

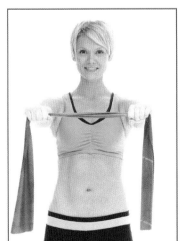

To Stretch or Not to Stretch

Sometimes stretching isn't the answer

Many people think if a muscle is tight, they should stretch it. This, however, is *not* always the case. Sometimes, muscles are tight because they are weak and they do not have enough strength or endurance to control the joint they are connected to, so, they hang on for dear life by spasming. Other times, the opposing muscle is overly strengthened and because of the imbalance, the weaker muscle spasms.

Spasm doesn't mean that the muscle twitches; it means that the muscle is holding a contraction. "Knots" in muscles are spasms, and many times when a muscle is tight it is because it is in spasm. If you stretch a muscle that is in spasm, often times it will relax and feel good, but once the body realizes that the muscle is relaxed and no longer protecting the joint, it will send the muscle back into spasm, sometimes worse than before. *In these situations, stretching doesn't help, it makes things worse!*

Strength over stretching

The best thing to do is *strengthen* the muscles surrounding the joint. The spasmed muscle needs some help! Strengthen that muscle so it can handle the workload put upon it, and help balance out the other muscles surrounding the joint.

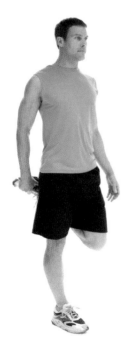

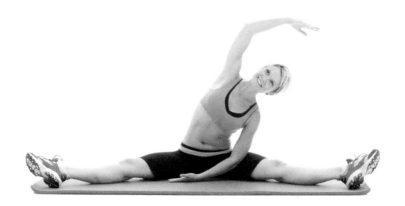

We're not saying that stretching is bad. We're just saying that sometimes it isn't the answer for tight muscles.

What is it and why is it important?

The "core" is a term thrown around by many trainers. But what exactly is it? Many people think that it's just your abs, but it's actually the musculature from the ribcage down through the hips. This is the central structure of the body, your gyroscope. If it's unbalanced, the rest of your body will be unbalanced as well.

Three important muscle groups in your abdomen:

1. **Rectus Abdominus**
   Your six-pack, controlling forward flexion of the body (bending forward in the mid-section)

2. **Internal and External Obliques**
   Your love-handle area. These muscles control your torso's rotation and side bending ability.

3. **Transverse Abdominus**
   The body girdle (or the weight belt). This is the deepest layer of abdominal muscle and it raps 360° around your torso from your hip bones to your ribs. This muscle controls the, "sucking in" motion of the abs and is one of the most important abdominal muscles in supporting the back and internal organs. *The proper activation of this muscle is the glue that connects and supports the entire abdominal system.*

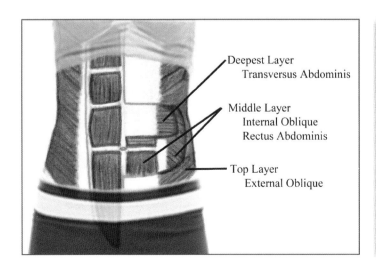

Deepest Layer
Transversus Abdominis

Middle Layer
Internal Oblique
Rectus Abdominis

Top Layer
External Oblique

Pull Your Abs IN

Many times, you may find yourself pushing your stomach out when contracting your abs. Not only does this fail to support your back, it will also make you look wide around the waistline. Activate the transverse muscle and pull in while doing all your exercises. This is the key to properly conditioning your core.

The Office Effect 10 Minute Exercise Program

IMPORTANT! FOR BEST RESULTS:

1. Do all the exercises in each exercise series and do them *in order* to employ *Counter Muscle Balancing*. This will ensure the best results.

2. *Switch it up.* Reverse the order every few weeks to avoid muscle adaptation.

3. Use *Wiggle, Bounce, and Roll* as warm-up before you exercises.

Upper Body Exercise Series

Chin Tucks	Seated Pullbacks
Huggers	Y-T Pulldowns
Servers	Hold-Ups
Offerings	Ski Jumpers

Designed to help *relieve*:

Numbness and Tingling (Hands)	Neck Pain
	Shoulder Pain
Headaches	Upper Back Pain

Designed to help *correct*:

Forward Head	Thoracic Outlet Syn
Hunched Shoulder	Rotated Head
Cervical Herniations	Lifted Shoulders

Lower Body Exercise Series

Perfect Crunches	Seated Twists
Swimmer Kicks	Double Leg Lifts
Marches	Clams
Bridges	Inner Thigh Leg Lifts

Designed to help *relieve*:

Numbness and Tingling (Feet)	Lower Back Pain
	Hip Pain
Sciatica	Groin Pain

Designed to help *correct*:

Rounded Lower Back	Lordosis
Raised Hip	SI Instability
Twisted Hips	Lumbar Herniations

Tummy Tuck-Ins

- Learn this exercise first, and then apply it to all the others.
- It will keep your body supported while performing all the exercises.
- It can make the difference between a flat belly and a pot belly.

Exercise Extras

Crossed Leg Twists	Press-Ups
Seated Clams	Ball Squeezes

Tummy Tuck-Ins

What this helps:

- Lower Back Pain (Lumbar Herniations)
- Rounded Lower Back

(20-30 Reps/Breaths)

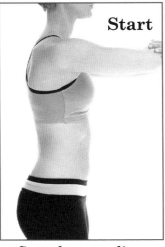

Start

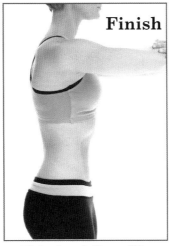

Finish

What you're working

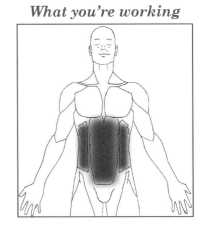

- Seated or standing, inhale while relaxing your abs.

- Exhale while pulling your belly button in and up.
- Hold for 3 to 5 seconds and repeat.

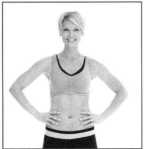

- To help you feel these muscles working, place your hands on either side of your waist while doing the exercise. You should feel your muscles tightening inward from your fingers and thumbs.

TIP: *To advance this exercise, see if you can keep your abs pulled in the whole time, even while inhaling.*

PAY ATTENTION TO:

** Use the Tummy Tuck-Ins with all other exercises to stabilize your core!

** Try to pull in from your rib cage down to your pubic bone.

** Fill your lungs up with air instead of your belly. This will allow you to have a deeper inward contraction.

** You can practice the Tummy Tuck-Ins while in your car or sitting at your desk.

DON'T DO THIS!

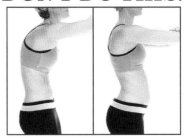

Avoid pushing your abs out and arching your lower back.

Chin Tucks

What this helps:
- Headaches and Neck Pain (Cervical Herniations)
- Forward Head

(15-25 Reps)

What you're working

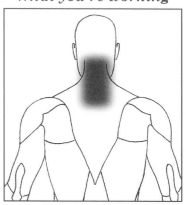

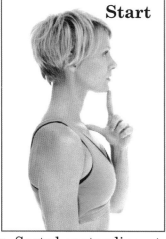 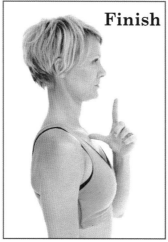

Start

Finish

- Seated or standing, start with your head and neck in their natural position.
- Place your hand in front of your neck with your thumb out and your index finger up.
- Your index finger touches the bottom of your chin in the starting position. *This will keep you from pushing your head forward.

- Gently pull your head straight back 1-2 inches.
- Release back to its normal position.

TIP: *It's great to do a few Chin Tucks throughout the day if you're staring at a computer for hours.*

DON'T DO THIS!

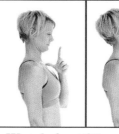 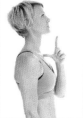

- Watch for tilting your head up or down.
- Don't pull back too hard.
- Watch for pushing your head forward when you release to your starting position.

PAY ATTENTION TO:
** Keep your movements slow and deliberate.
** Try putting a Chin Tucks reminder on your desk or computer.
** You may also hold your head in the back position for 1-3 seconds before releasing it back to your starting position.

What this helps:

- Shoulder Pain
- *Allows you to work with a keyboard and mouse for longer periods of times*

(10-15 Reps)

Start

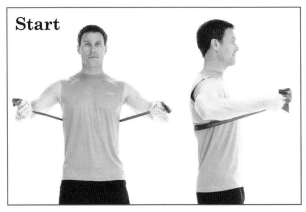

- Stand or sit with your elbows bent and out to the side, just below shoulder height, shoulders relaxed.
- Have the red band in both hands and wrapped around your back, or around the back of a chair if you're seated.
- Elbows should be straight out from your torso.

Finish

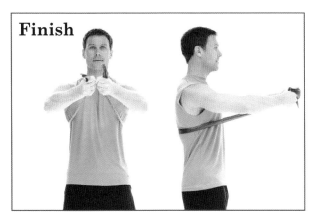

- Exhale while pulling your abs in and pressing your arms out until your knuckles touch.
- Inhale while slowly returning to the start position.

What you're working

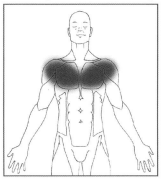

TIP: *It's like you're hugging a beach ball.*

DON'T DO THIS!

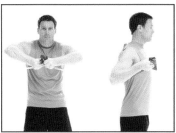

- Don't lift your shoulders.
- Don't flair your ribcage by pulling your elbows behind your back.

PAY ATTENTION TO:

** Keep your chin up.
** Don't lean back while pressing your arms forward.
** Don't round your upper back by over extending your arms forward.
** Keep your elbows from dropping.

What this helps:
- Upper Back Pain
- Hunched Shoulder

(10-15 Reps)

What you're working

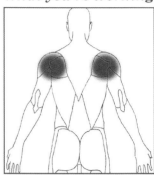

TIP: *Pretend your elbows are glued to your side.*

Start

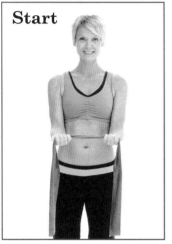

Finish

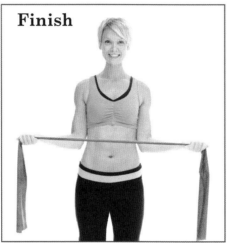

- Sit in a chair or stand.
- Relax your shoulders down, squeeze your arms against your side, make sure your elbows are slightly in front.
- Hold the band in both hands with a tiny bit of slack, palms facing upward, hands a few inches apart, and elbows bent at 90°.

- Exhale as you simultaneously rotate both hands outward until they reach a "V" shape from your torso. Your elbows should stay glued to your side.
- Inhale as you slowly return to your starting position.

DON'T DO THIS!

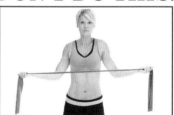

- Don't lift your shoulders.
- Don't allow your arms to pull away from your side or your elbows to slide behind your torso.

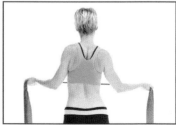

- Watch pinching your shoulder blades together.

PAY ATTENTION TO:
** Keep from bending elbows more than 90°.
** These are small stabilizing muscles, so you may not feel them until the 3rd or 4th rep.
** Sometimes, you may feel as if the work is coming from the middle of your arm, this is OK.
** If you have really tight chest muscles, you may even feel them stretch.

What this helps:

- Shoulder Pain
- *Allows you to work with a keyboard and mouse for longer periods of time*

(10-15 Reps)

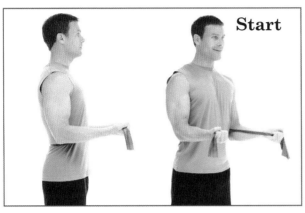

Start

- Standing or seated, have the band in both hands and around your back or the back of a chair.
- Shoulders down, elbows by your side, palms facing up and holding the band.

TIP: *Imagine you're offering a heavy tray of food to someone.*

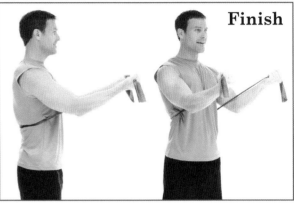

Finish

- Exhale, engaging your abs while pressing your hands forward and up until they almost reach shoulder height, but no higher.
- Be sure to keep your shoulders down and your elbows facing down toward the floor.
- Inhale as you bend your elbows back to starting position.

What you're working

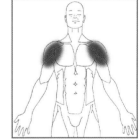

PAY ATTENTION TO:

** Don't fully straighten your arms.
** Keep your palms facing up throughout the exercise.
** Use your abs to keep your rib cage from flaring.
** Check your posture and make sure you are sitting up straight or standing straight throughout the exercise.

DON'T DO THIS!

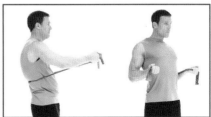

- Watch leaning back.
- Don't lift or hunch your shoulders.
- Don't allow your elbows to pass your torso on the return to start position.

Seated Pullbacks

What this helps:
- Upper Back and Shoulder Pain
- Hunched Shoulders

(10-15 Reps)

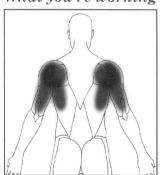

What you're working

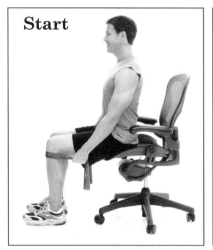

Start

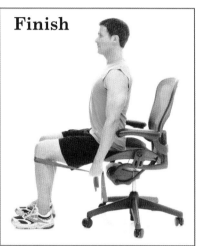

Finish

- Sitting on the edge of your chair, knees hip distance apart.
- Place the band around your knees, hold in both hands a few inches behind your knees, palms facing inward toward your legs.

- Gently reach your arms toward the floor by activating the muscles under your armpits.
- Exhale as you pull your arms back, until they line up with your torso.
- Inhale as you slowly return to the start position, continuing to feel the work in the back of your arms, and keeping the gentle pull down in your shoulders.

DON'T DO THIS!

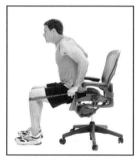

- Don't raise your shoulders or pinch your shoulder blades together.

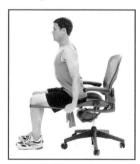

- Don't stick your chest out.
- Don't pull your arms past your torso.

> *TIP: Keep your chest open by imagining you have a big smile ☺ from shoulder to shoulder.*

PAY ATTENTION TO:
** Keep your wrists straight.
** Don't lean forward as you pull your arms back.
** If you feel pain in your neck, you probably have too much tension on your band.

What this helps:
- Upper Shoulder and Neck Pain
- Lifted Shoulders

(10-15 Reps)

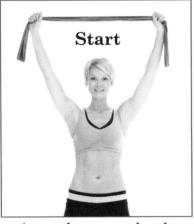

Start

- Arms above your head, shoulders down with a wide back.
- Hold the band in your hands about 2 feet apart, palms facing forward.

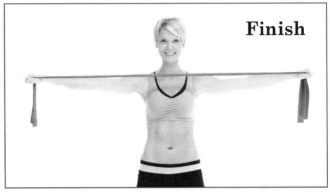

Finish

- Exhale as you gently pull your ribs and abs in, while pulling your arms out and down, until they are in line with your shoulders. Make sure the band goes just in front of your nose.
- Inhale while returning your arms slowly to their starting position. Work to keep your shoulders down as you return to your starting position.

What you're working

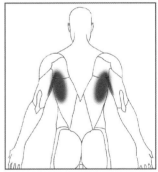

TIP: *Use your abs! Pulling them in will prevent you from pushing your rib cage out.*

PAY ATTENTION TO:
** Keep your arms even with each other.
** If this exercise is too easy, you can always double up the band by folding it in half.
** If you can't open your arms all the way down to your shoulders, your band may be too tight. Add some slack in the band before you begin the pulldown.

DON'T DO THIS!

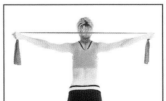

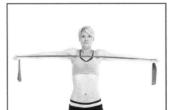

- Be careful not to pinch your shoulder blades together.
- Don't pull the band behind your head.

- Don't lift your shoulders.
- Don't push your ribs out.

What this helps:

- Neck and Upper Back Pain
- Hunched Shoulders and Forward Head (Postural Kyphosis)

(Hold 15 to 60 Secs)

Start

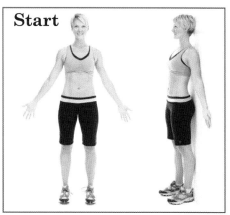

Finish
(Version 1)

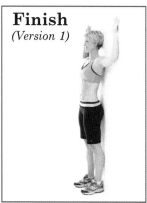

Finish
(Version 2)

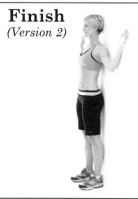

Note: You only need to do one version, so pick whichever one works for you.

- Stand against a wall with your heels, buttocks, shoulders, hands, and the back of your head against it.
- With your palms facing out, move your arms out at a slight angle.

- Exhale while drawing your bellybutton toward your spine and bend your elbows.
- Slide your arms up the wall until your elbows are in line with your shoulders (make sure your shoulders are not lifted). Hold for 15-60 seconds.

- Slide the back of your hands up the wall until they are even or slightly higher than your shoulders, keeping your mid/upper back, shoulders, and hands in contact with the wall. Hold for 15-60 seconds.

What you're working

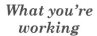
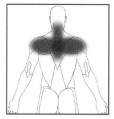

TIP: *This is a stand-alone exercise. If you only have a minute, and you've been sitting at your desk for hours, this is a great exercise to do.*

PAY ATTENTION TO:

** Use your abs (Tummy Tuck-Ins) to keep your mid-back from lifting off the wall.
** Use a mirror to make sure your arms are the same height.
** Keep your head against the wall, without raising your chin.
** If your hands move off the wall, that's OK, don't force it.

DON'T DO THIS!

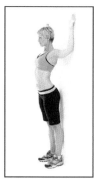

- Don't raise your shoulders.
- Don't lift your mid-back off the wall.
- Don't pinch your shoulder blades together.

Ski Jumpers

What this helps:

- Back, Neck, and Shoulder Pain
- Forward Head, Hunched Shoulders, and Rounded Lower Back
  (Thoracic Herniations and Postural Kyphosis)

(10-15 Reps)
hold for 3-5 seconds each

Start

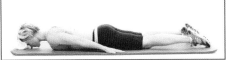

- Lie flat on your stomach, arms by your side, palms facing down, legs together and straight, head resting in natural position with your forehead on a small towel.

Advanced Finish
(Feet Up)

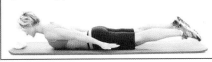

- Lift your legs a few inches off the ground when you lift your upper body. Keep your legs straight and your feet pointed. This will engage your buttocks and hamstrings.

Finish

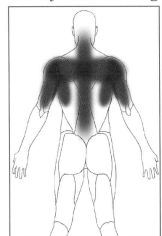

- Exhale as you pull in your abs and gently lift your head and chest off the floor just a few inches. At the same time, lift your arms and hands off the floor and gently pull them down toward your feet. Hold for 3-5 seconds.
- Keep your eyes focused on a spot six inches in front of you to maintain proper neck alignment.
- Inhale as you return to your starting position.

What you're working

TIP: *Imagine you're flying through the air, catching the wind with your hands.*

PAY ATTENTION TO:

** Lifting your back too high can hurt your back.
** Feel as if your neck is pulling out from your shoulders and your back is lengthening, not compressing.
** Keep legs on the floor unless you're doing the advanced version.

DON'T DO THIS!

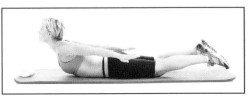

- Don't lift your chin or pull your head back.
- Don't pinch your shoulder blades together.
- Watch dropping your head down.

Perfect Crunches

What this helps:

- Lower Back Pain
- Arched Lower Back
  (Lumbar Herniations and Lordosis)

As many reps as possible

Start

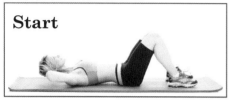

- Lie on your back, knees bent, feet flat on the floor, hip distance apart.
- Fingers intertwined and behind your head, elbows wide.
- Keep your head and neck completely relaxed in your hands and your eyes gazing straight up at the ceiling.
- Lift your head and shoulders just one inch off the ground by contracting your abs in.

Finish

- Exhale while pulling your ribs in and down toward your hips by further engaging your abs and pulling your bellybutton toward your spine.
- This should cause your head and shoulders to lift another 1-2 inches off the floor (keep looking at the ceiling).
- Inhale while returning to your starting position with your head and shoulders floating one inch off the floor and your abs still engaged.

What you're working

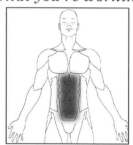

TIP: *Pull your abs IN and keep them engaged at all times during this exercise (even when returning to starting position). This is the key!*

Advanced Finish
(Feet Up)

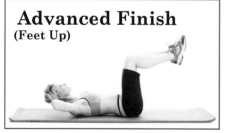

- Be sure to maintain a slight curve in your lower back.

PAY ATTENTION TO:

** Keeping the natural curve in your lower back is very important.

** Try and fill your back with air (using your lungs) instead of your diaphragm (filling your belly with air). This will greatly help you pull in your abs.

** Place a small rolled up towel under your lower back to help it keep its natural curve.

DON'T DO THIS!

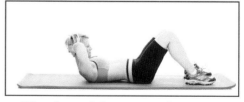

- Watch pushing your abs out instead of pulling them in.
- Don't pull your chin into your chest or pull on your neck.
- Keep from pressing your lower back into the floor.
- Don't roll your hips under (your legs should be relaxed).

What this helps:
- Lower Back and Hip Pain
  (Lumbar Herniations, SI Instability, Sciatica)
- Rounded Lower Back

(10-15 Reps) Per Leg

Start

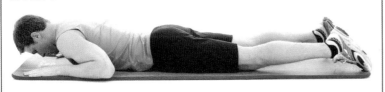

- Lie flat on your stomach, hands on floor, abs pulled in.
- Shoulders gently pulling down toward your feet, head resting on a small towel.
- Feet pointed with legs slightly turned out, about hip distance apart.

What you're working

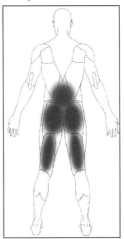

Finish

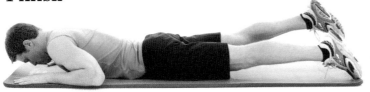

- Exhale while pulling your abs in, lift one leg a few inches off the floor with a pointed foot. Keep legs straight.
- Inhale while returning your leg to the start position.
- Repeat with the opposite leg.

***TIP**: Try this exercise with a pillow under your hips for better range of motion.*

PAY ATTENTION TO:
** Use your abs to stabilize your hips so they don't rock back and forth.
** Squeeze your thigh muscle to keep your leg straight.
** To advance this exercise, keep both legs slightly off the ground while simultaneously switching legs (scissoring) in a slow rhythm.

DON'T DO THIS!

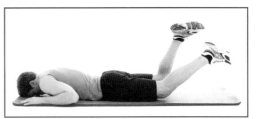

- Don't lift legs more than 3-6 inches off the floor.
- Don't bend legs at the knee.
- Don't shrug shoulders.
- *If your back starts hurting, you're probably lifting your legs too high.*

What this helps:
- Lower Back and Hip Pain
  (Lumbar Herniations, SI Instability, Sciatica)
- Rounded Lower Back

(10-15 Reps) Per Leg

Start

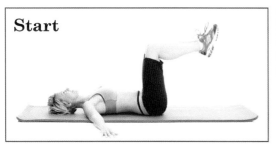

- Lie on your back, arms by your side, shoulders relaxed and down, lower back in its natural curve.
- Pull your abs in to lift one leg at a time, until you reach the starting position with both legs in the air, knees bent at 90°. *Be sure not to increase the small arch in your lower back when lifting your legs.*

TIP: *It is normal to feel this exercise in your thighs, hips, and lower back, but the key is to get most of the work in your lower abs instead.*

Finish

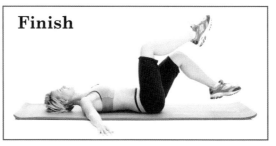

- Exhale while pulling your abs in and slowly lower one foot toward the floor (maintaining the 90° angle of your knee).
- Gently tap your toe on the floor.
- Inhale and continue engaging your abs as you bring your leg back up to starting position.
- Repeat with your other leg.
- *Note: If your lower back gets tight during this exercise, try flattening your lower back (just don't smash your back into the ground).*

What you're working

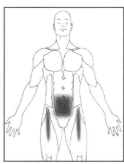

PAY ATTENTION TO:
** Try to relax your hip flexors (front crease of your hip) and work your lower abs.
** Keep legs and knees in alignment with your hips.
** If your lower back starts to hurt, you may be reaching too far with your foot or you're not concentrating on using your abs.
** Focus your attention on pulling in, 2 inches below your bellybutton.

DON'T DO THIS!

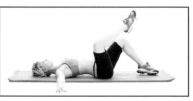

- Don't over arch your lower back. If this is happening, reconnect with your abs.
- Avoid tensing your neck and shoulders.
- Don't let your knees open up to the side.

Bridges

What this helps:

- Tight Hamstrings (back of legs), Glutes (buttocks), Lower Back, and Hip Pain (Lumbar Herniations, SI Instability, Sciatica)
- Rounded Lower Back

(15-20 Reps)

What you're working

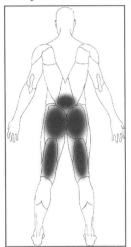

Start

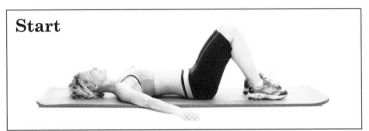

- Lie on your back, arms by your side, knees bent, feet flat on the floor, hip distance apart, about 1 foot from your buttocks.

Finish

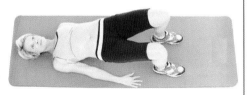

- Exhale as you press into your feet, keeping your entire foot in contact with the floor, to lift your hips about 6-8 inches.
- Inhale as you bring your hips back down to the floor.
- When you lift, keep the same curve in your lower back as you had when you started.

: If it starts to hurt your lower back, you may be going too high or arching your back too much.

DON'T DO THIS!

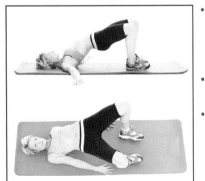

- Don't roll your hips up or round your lower back.
- Don't roll your feet in or out.
- Watch out for over arching your back at the top of the lift.

PAY ATTENTION TO:

** Keep your knees parallel.
** Keep your neck and shoulders relaxed.
** If you are not feeling it in your glutes, you may not be lifting high enough. Squeeze your butt!

What this helps:
- Lower Back and Hip Pain
- Lifted and Rotated Hips
- *Counters torso rotations you do throughout the day and helps prevent disc herniations*

(10-15 Reps) Per Side

What you're working

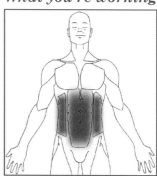

Start

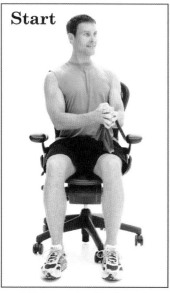

Finish

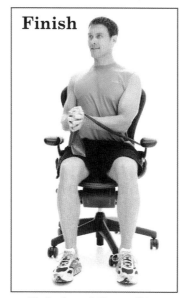

- Sit in a chair, feet flat on the floor, with band wrapped around one armrest.
- Grasp the band with both hands.
- Keep your elbows pressed against your torso and bent at 90°.
- If possible, have enough tension on the band so that your torso is slightly rotated toward the armrest that the band is wrapped around.

- Exhale while pulling your abs in and up to elongate your spine while simultaneously rotating your torso to the other side of the chair.
- Inhale while rotating your torso back to the starting position, without losing the lift and connection to your abs.

Note: *This exercise can be done standing with the band attached to a doorknob.*

TIP: Imagine you're like a corkscrew. As you rotate, your spine lengthens as it spirals upward.

DON'T DO THIS!

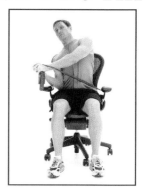

- Don't lift your hip as you rotate.
- Don't lean back as you rotate.
- Avoid lifting your shoulders and flaring out your elbows.

PAY ATTENTION TO:
** This is an ab exercise. If you're feeling it in your shoulders or back, your arms may not be glued to your body.
** Remember to use the Tummy Tuck-Ins with this exercise.

Double Leg Lifts

What this helps:
- Lower Back, Hip, and Groin Pain (SI Instability)
- Lifted Hip

(10-15 Reps) Per Side

Start

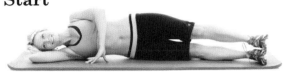

- Lie on your side, your bottom arm (or pillow) supporting your head, your legs straight with both legs stacked on top of each other.
- From the top of your head to your feet should be one straight line.
- Your top arm is in front of your body with your palm on the floor for balance.
- Pull in and secure your abs.

Finish

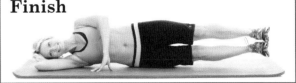

- Exhale while continuing to pull in your abs as you lift both legs simultaneously, about 3-6 inches off the floor.
- Inhale as you lower your legs back to the floor (starting position) while still pulling in your abs.
- For an added challenge, keep both legs floating one inch off the floor when you return to the start position.

TIP: When you practice this exercise, switch which side you start on every time you do it.

What you're working

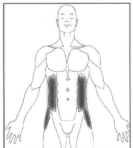

PAY ATTENTION TO:
** If you feel this exercise in your back, allow your top hip to rotate backward an inch or two and keep that hip placement throughout the exercise.
** Remember your Tummy Tuck-Ins throughout the entire exercise.
** You can also place your top arm on your hip, which challenges your balance.
** If you are having balance problems or you feel this exercise in your back, try to have your legs 4-6 in front of you throughout the exercise.

DON'T DO THIS!

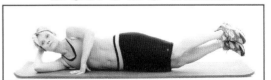

- Don't roll your top hip bone forward.
- Watch tensing your neck and shoulders.
- Don't lift your head.
- Be careful not to lift your legs too high.

What this helps:

- Lower Back, Hip, Groin, and Glute (buttocks) Pain (Lumbar Herniations, SI Instability, Sciatica)
- Lifted and Rotated Hips

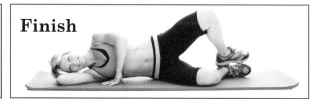

(15-20 Reps)
Per Side

Start

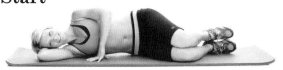

- Lie on your side with your head, shoulders, hips and feet in a line, head supported by your arm or pillow. Make sure your knees are bent and just below waist level.
- Heels are together, lower back in its natural curve. Hips are stacked on top of each other, you're not leaning back or forward with your top hip. (If your top knee isn't in line with your bottom knee then your hips aren't aligned properly either.)

Finish

- Pulling your abs in, exhale as you lift your top knee up as high as it can go while keeping your top hip bone from moving.
- Inhale as you return to your starting position.
- To help your hips stay level, try placing a small, rolled up towel under your waist.

What you're working

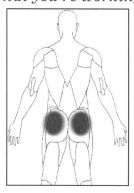

TIP: *If you have stiff or painful shoulders, use a pillow or rolled up towel to support your head.*

DON'T DO THIS!

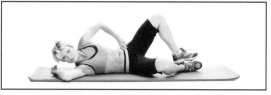

- Don't rock your top hip back.
- Don't open your legs in a fast or jerky motion.

PAY ATTENTION TO:

** Keep your abs engaged the entire time to prevent your hips from wobbling.
** Relax your neck and shoulders.
** When you practice this exercise, switch which side you start on every time you do it.
** There should be no movement in your hips.

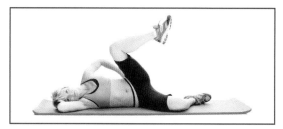

- Try not to separate your heels as you lift your knees.

What this helps:

- Lower Back, Hip, and Groin Pain
  (Lumbar Herniation, SI Instability, Sciatica)
- Lifted and Twisted Hips

**(15-20 Reps)
Per Side**

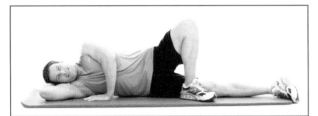

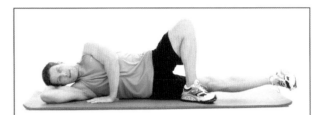

- Lie on your side with your bottom arm or pillow supporting your head, your body in a straight line.
- Cross your top leg over your bottom leg with your foot flat on the floor.
- Your top arm should be in front of your body with your palm on the floor to support yourself.
- Your top hip should be slightly tilted back.
- Your bottom leg should be straight with tension in your thigh.

- Pulling in on your abs, exhale as you lift your bottom leg 2-4 inches off the ground.
- Inhale as you lower your leg back down toward the floor, but do not let it fully rest on the floor (keep your leg floating one inch off the floor).
- Repeat the exercise.

What you're working

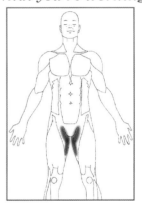

TIP: *In many cases, working your inner thigh muscles can greatly reduce lower back pain.*

PAY ATTENTION TO:

** Use your abs to control hip wiggling.
** Keep it slow and smooth; don't jerk your leg.
** When you practice this exercise, switch which side you start on every time.
** To advance this exercise, do little circles and reverse circles with your working leg, but make sure you really hold in your abs so your hips don't start wiggling.

DON'T DO THIS!

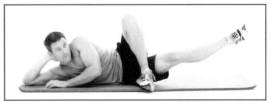

- Avoid rolling your top hip bone too far backward.
- Try not to tense or lift your neck.
- Don't bend the leg you're lifting.

Crossed Leg Twists
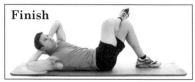

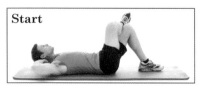

(15-20 Reps) Per Side

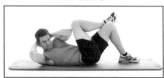

Don't

- Fingers intertwined behind your head, elbows wide, one leg crossed.
- Relax neck, gazing straight up at ceiling.
- Lift head and shoulders just one inch off the ground by contracting abs in.
- Keep a small curve in your lower back throughout the exercise.

- Keeping your gaze on the ceiling, exhale, rotating slightly to one side, keeping shoulders and head off the floor.
- Inhale, returning to start position with head and shoulders staying a few inches off the floor, abs continually engaged.
- After full reps, switch legs and direction.

- Don't pull chin to chest.
- Don't pull elbow to knee.
- Don't flatten lower back.
- Don't release abdominal contraction at any time.

Seated Clams
(w/ Red Band)

Clams alternative

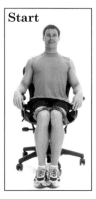
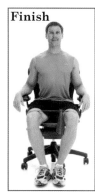

(10-15 Reps)

Start:
- Seated in a chair, legs at 90°, knees and feet together, band tied around thighs (not too tight).

Finish:
- Exhale while pulling your abs in and separating both legs simultaneously, making sure they are opening at equal distances.
- Inhale while returning to the starting position.

Don't
- Don't lean or hunch forward.
- Make sure the band is close to your knees.
- Don't round your lower back.

Note:
If it's too easy, wrap the band around your legs twice.

Press-Ups

lower back herniation repair

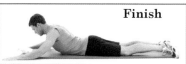

(15-20 Reps)

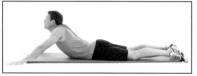

Don't

- Lying on your stomach, elbows straight out from shoulders, hands flat on the floor.
- Head facing straight down, forehead on towel, legs hip distance apart, slightly turned out.

- With your abs RELAXED, slowly press into your hands, using your arm strength to raise your upper body 6 inches to a foot off the floor.
- Keep your neck and head in line with your back.
- Keep your shoulders sliding down toward your hips as you press up.

- Don't press up too high, this is a gentle, passive back bend.
- Keep shoulders down.
- Don't pinch shoulder blades together.
- Don't look down at floor.
- Don't fully straighten arms.

*Inner Thigh
Leg Lifts alternative*

Ball Squeezes

(10-15 Reps)

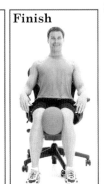

Start | Finish

Start:
- Place a ball between your knees while sitting in a chair.
- Be sure to have your feet parallel and don't round your lower back in your chair.
- Sit toward edge of seat, lean back, keeping the curve in your lower back. Support your body with arms on your arm rests.

Finish:
- Exhale while squeezing your knees together, holding for a few seconds, then release.

Don't
- Make sure your feet are hip distance apart.
- Don't hunch or lean forward.

Note:
If you hear or feel a pop in your groin area, don't be alarmed, you didn't break anything. It is probably your pubis resetting itself, kind of like popping a knuckle.

Fast Relief

Although our exercise series are specifically designed to employ *Counter Muscle Balancing*, there are a few exercises that can be done by themselves if you only have a few minutes. These are OK if you're in a pinch, and they can give you some immediate relief, but if you want to *fix it for life*, you should do the full series.

Area of Pain	Exercise
Lower Back	Ball Squeezes
Lower Back	Tummy Tuck-Ins
Neck & Headaches	Chin Tucks
Upper Shoulders & Stress	Y-T Pulldowns
Upper Back & Shoulders	Hold-Ups
Neck, Upper & Lower Back	Ski Jumpers

Quick Reference Guide

Area Of Pain	Postural Conditions	Environmental Causes	How to Fix It	Exercise & Quick Relief
Neck Headaches Tingling/Numbness in Fingers	Forward Head Raised Shoulders	Monitor too far away Keyboard too high Chair too low	Move monitor closer Keyboard at bellybutton Raise chair Raise armrests	Upper Body Series *Chin Tucks
One Side of Neck (movement based)	Rotated Head Tilted Head Lifted Shoulder	Mouse too far away Monitor in corner Transcribing document off to side and/or low	Move mouse closer Center monitor Raise/center documents	Upper Body Series *Chin Tucks *Y-T Pulldowns
One Shoulder	Raised Shoulder Hunched Shoulder	Mouse too far away Armrests too low Pinching phone between head & shoulder	Move mouse closer Raise armrests Use Headset	Upper Body Series *Y-T Pulldowns *Servers
Upper Trap Shoulders	Raised Shoulders Hunched Shoulders Forward Head	Monitor too far away Chair too low Keyboard too far away Keyboard too high Armrests too low	Move monitor closer Raise chair Move keyboard closer Keyboard at bellybutton Raise armrests	Upper Body Series *Y-T Pulldowns *Chin Tucks *Servers
Chest Upper Back	Forward Head Hunched Shoulders Rounded Upper Back	Monitor too far away Keyboard too far away Mouse too far away	Move monitor closer Keyboard at bellybutton Move mouse closer	Upper Body Series *Ski Jumpers
Lower Back	Rounded Lower Back Rotated Torso Crossed Leg Weight on one Leg/Hip	No lumbar support Phone, fax, file cabinet off to one side	Use lumbar support Use swivel chair Sit/stand with equal weight on both hips/legs	Lower Body Series *Ball Squeezes *Swimmer Kicks
Hip Buttocks Groin	Rounded Lower Back Rotated Torso Weight on one Leg/Hip Crossed Leg	No lumbar support Phone, fax, file cabinet off to one side	Use lumbar support Use swivel chair Sit/stand with equal weight on both hips/legs Don't cross legs or switch legs periodically	Lower Body Series *Clams *Inner Thigh Leg Lifts *Twists
Sciatica	Rounded Lower Back Crossed Leg Weight on one Leg/Hip	No lumbar support Phone, fax, file cabinet off to one side	Use lumbar support Don't cross legs or switch legs periodically Sit/stand with equal weight on both hips/legs	Lower Body Series *Swimmer Kicks *Clams and Inner Thigh Leg Lifts
Carpal Tunnel	Bent Wrists Hunched Shoulders Forward Head	No wrist support Chair too low Keyboard too high Monitor too far away Armrest too low	Use wrist supports Raise chair Keyboard at bellybutton Move monitor closer Raise armrests	Upper Body Series *Median Nerve Stretch

Part V
Fix It
Outside the Office

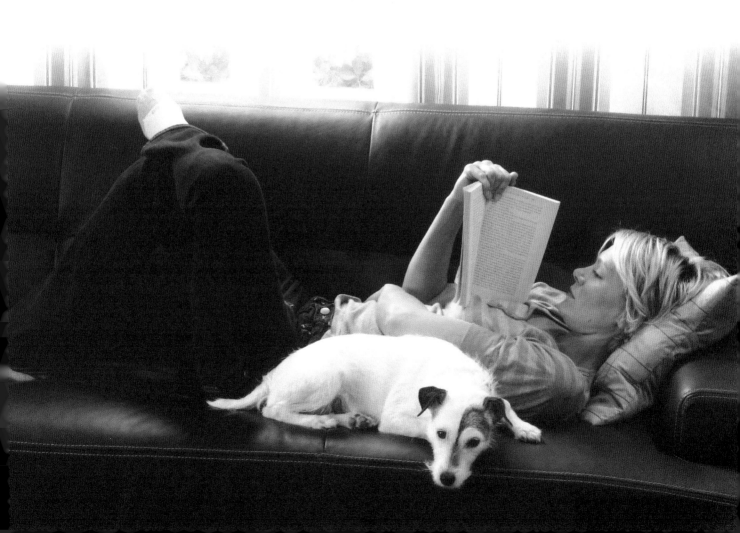

True Stories of *The Office Effect*

Client Story #2: Twist and Shout

One of my clients came to me and she was twisted, literally. Her right hip was lifted and rotated forward, causing her upper torso to face one way and her hips to face another. She was experiencing pain in her lower back and hip. I first asked if she had been in an accident or had any injuries and she said, "No." Without an inciting incident for her twist, I knew it was probably a repetitive stress that was causing her pain and body rotation. I had a good idea that it had to be something she was doing on a daily basis to cause such a noticeable problem. Since most people spend the majority of their time at work, I knew that would be a good place to start looking for the possible cause. So I asked her what a typical day at the office was like. She said she spent most of her time at her desk, receiving phone calls and faxes because she worked in a billing department. I had a hunch so I asked about how many faxes she received per day. She said, "Around forty to fifty." I then asked where her fax machine was located. She said it was at the back right corner of her desk. Finally, I asked if she had a swivel chair. She replied, "No." I smiled, knowing that we had found the cause of her twist and pain.

Because her chair didn't swivel, she had to twist her body to the right forty to fifty times a day, five days a week, in order to grab the incoming faxes. That's as many as one thousand repetitions a month—and she had been doing this job for over six months. This caused her to continually contract the rotational muscles of her torso, but only on the right side of her body. So the right side became over developed, pulling and twisting her hips off and causing her pain.

I had her get a swivel chair so she no longer rotated her body and instead rotated the chair. I then had her do a rotation exercise to work her obliques, called the Seated Twists, but only to the left for a few weeks to combat all the right side rotations she had been doing for months. After that, I gave her *The Office Effect 10 Minute Exercise Program* so she could keep her body balanced, no matter what she happened to do at work. In one month, her twist was gone and she was out of pain.

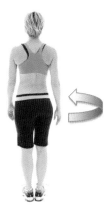

> *"The 3 F's Method is a much healthier solution to my neck and shoulder pain than pain pills and expensive treatments. Plus, I feel like I'm healing myself."*
>
> *Anita,*
> *Client*

The Office Effect at Home

The Office Effect doesn't just happen at the office; it can also happen as a result of the things we do at home and in our everyday lives. Just like sitting at a desk can change your posture and cause pain, the duties that you perform around the house can have the same impact. Fortunately, *The 3 F's Method* can be applied almost anywhere.

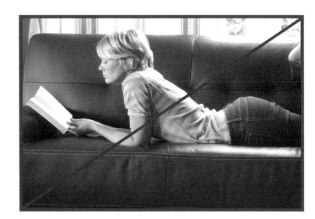

Identify the aches and pains that come with a day of cleaning, shopping, playing with the kids, and trying to keep a household together. Put your detective hat on and begin to look for the repetitive stresses that lurk throughout the house.

When you feel pain, take the time to acknowledge it rather than just ignore it. Then make the decision to live your life as pain free as possible and make the necessary adjustments.

Be a Repetitive Stress Detective

In this section, you will see some of the most common scenarios for painful repetitive stresses outside the office. Compare these scenarios to your own life and note the similarities. Be aware of what these everyday activities can do to your body over time if you don't address them.

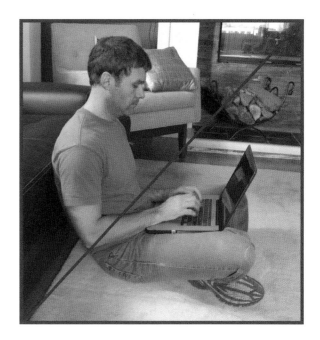

Remember, repetitive stress is a fact of life, and no matter how diligent you are, you will never be able to eliminate it from your life completely. However, you don't have to let it change your body and bring you down. Once you develop an awareness of these potentially harmful repetitive stresses, you will see that the solutions require very little effort, but can make a very big difference in how you look and feel.

Vacuuming

Believe it or not, this activity can easily cause lower back pain, SI joint (hip) instability, and shoulder pain, especially if you have a heavy vacuum or a high pile rug.

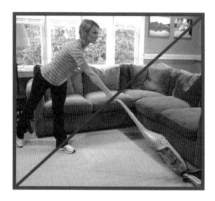 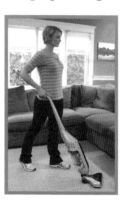

✓ **Limit your range of motion when pushing the vacuum back and forth.**
✓ **Keep your elbow facing down toward the floor.**
✓ **Consciously hold your abs in (Tummy Tuck-Ins).**
✓ **Switch sides periodically.**
✓ *The Office Effect* **Upper Body Exercise Series will help with pain caused by vacuuming.**

Laundry

I actually had an Olympic gold medalist as a client who had a lower back herniation she sustained while doing laundry...laundry! It is a common occurrence, and it's the result of bending over to get the laundry out of the basket, then lifting while twisting to place it in the machine.

✓ **Place your laundry basket on a chair so you don't have to bend over to get the clothes out of the basket and put them into the machine.**
✓ **Place the basket directly in front of the machine to prevent twisting.**

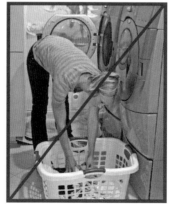 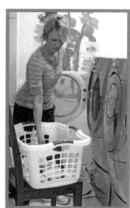

Cleaning Counters

Reaching across counters and cleaning in large, circular motions can cause the muscles in your shoulder to spasm from overwork. You may also experience pain in one side of your lower back, especially if your hips are not centered while cleaning.

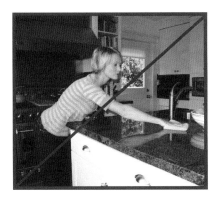 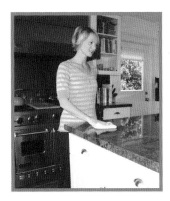

✓ **Keep your arm close to the body when you clean, try not to overextend your arm.**
✓ **Keep your elbow down toward the floor.**
✓ **Consciously hold your abs in while cleaning (Tummy Tuck-Ins).**
✓ **Periodically switch the direction of your cleaning to balance the shoulder muscles better.**
✓ **Continually switch arms while cleaning.**
✓ **Make sure your hips and torso are directly facing the surface you're cleaning.**
✓ ***The Office Effect* Upper Body Exercise Series will help with pain caused by cleaning counters.**

Brushing Your Teeth

Brushing your teeth...really? If you have a lower back herniation or pain and stiffness, then brushing your teeth can be a hazard. This is because most people lean over the sink while they brush, causing the lower back muscles to strain as they keep you from falling head first into the mirror. This can cause the lower back muscles to spasm or a herniation to bulge further, all of which cause pain.

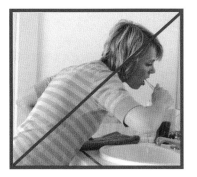 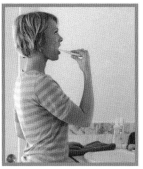

✓ **Pretty simple fix, don't lean over the sink the entire time you are brushing.**
✓ **Also, drop your elbow down toward the floor on the arm that you brush with. This will help reduce the strain on your shoulder muscles.**

Holding Children

Many of our clients who have small children complain of lower back, shoulder, and hip pain. This usually occurs because they rest their child on one of their hips, and then hike that hip up in order to support their child. This will cause the muscles surrounding the hip and lower back on that side to overwork, becoming unbalanced as they support the trunk of the body.

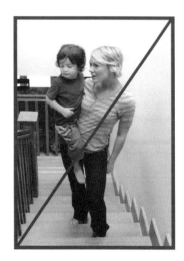
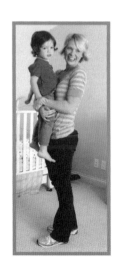

- ✓ **If you must hold your child on the side, do not hike your hip up. Use your arm strength and keep your shoulder down and your elbow close to your body.**
- ✓ **Switch the side you're holding your child on periodically.**
- ✓ **Hold your child in front of your body, not on one hip.**
- ✓ **Most importantly, EXERCISE! Carrying around a ten to thirty pound child all day while trying to do things is simply going to put a strain on your body. Do *The Office Effect* Upper and Lower Body Exercise Series consistently, so that you can handle the strain.**

Playing with Children

The most taxing thing about playing with your child is that you're usually hunched over on the ground to be at their level as you race the cars around the track or dress up dolls. This can put a strain on your lower and upper back because you can't maintain a proper posture while playing with things on the ground.

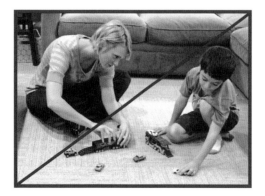
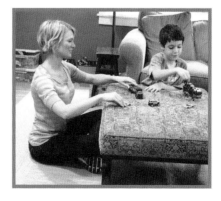

- ✓ **Raise the playing surface. Place the toys on a table, a footstool, or ottoman. Then you can sit or kneel on the floor with a pillow under your hips that will allow you to maintain proper posture and reduce the strain on your back.**

Picking Up a Child

Most parents bend at the waist with straight legs, reaching away from their body with their elbows out as they lift their child up. This puts a strain on the back, hips, hamstrings, and shoulders causing herniations, strains, and spasms.

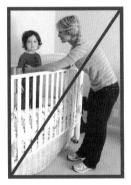 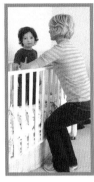 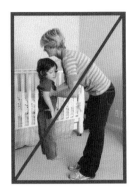 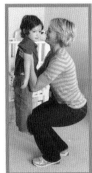

✓ **The best way to lift your child is to face them straight on. Have them close to your body, with your knees bent, and your lower back in its natural curve (don't be rounded or hunched over).**
✓ **Lift on an exhale, keeping your elbows close to the body and using your legs to stand up.**

Cleaning Up after the Kids

You're just picking up toys that weigh less than a pound, but that's all it takes to injure yourself. Many parents come to us in pain as they feel a pop in their back from simply picking up a toy.

✓ **Grab a bin and get down on the floor so you don't have to strain your back by bending over.**

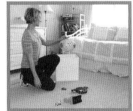

Kids Need Good Posture Too

The way these two kids are sitting on the couch can put undue stress on their necks. They are still growing, and if this is a continual postural pattern, it can cause their spine, ligaments, tendons, and muscles to develop in an unnatural and destructive way.

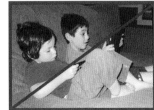

✓ **Keep an eye on the little ones. If you show them proper posture now, they'll have a head start on staying healthy and keeping themselves out of pain.**

Lounging

The couch is a spine killer, causing neck, upper back, and lower back pain. It can cause tingling in the hands and feet, Sciatica, and headaches as well. As you're zoned into your favorite TV show, you don't always notice the pain that is starting in your neck until you stand up and realize your arm is numb. Since the couch lacks lumbar support and is so squishy, holding a proper posture is next to impossible. So, how do you fix it?

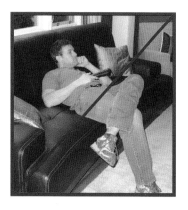
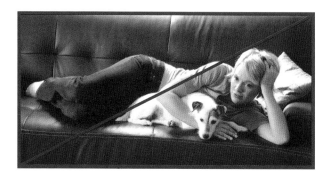

- ✓ **Sit up on the couch instead of lying on your side.**
- ✓ **Place a pillow under your lower back to help maintain the curve in your lower back.**
- ✓ **Limit propping your legs up on an ottoman. This will stretch the hamstrings and round the lower back.**
- ✓ **The height of your TV should be at eye level to avoid straining the neck.**

Walking the Dog

I know the dog trainer told you that Spike has to be on your left side every time you walk him but your trainer wasn't thinking about your body. Your dog may pull you during walks and you may end up overworking or straining the muscles on just one side of your body, especially if you walk your dog on the same side every time.

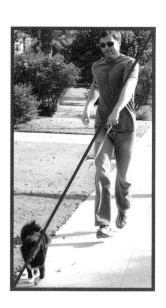

- ✓ **Switch which side you walk your dog on every day.**
- ✓ **Keep the leash close to your body.**
- ✓ **Doing *The Office Effect* Upper and Lower Body Exercise Series can help you be strong throughout your entire body, just in case Spike finds a squirrel he'd like to chase.**

On the Phone, In the Car

Talking on the Phone

If you have your head cocked to one side, pinching your phone between your shoulder and ear, you can do a number on your neck muscles and cervical spine. A two-minute call can cause your neck muscles to spasm and put you in pain.

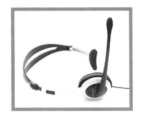

✓ **Get a headset or earpiece.**

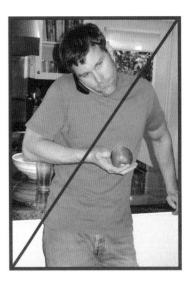

Proper Car Posture

The days of ten and two o'clock hand positions on the wheel are over. If you have a long commute to work every day, you can do some serious damage to your body. You may not be able to obtain the same optimal sitting position in your car as you can at your desk but there is a whole lot you can do to help.

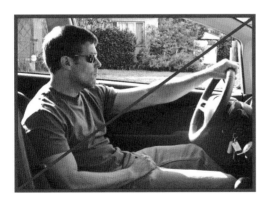
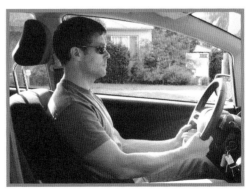

✓ **Make sure your seat back is up so your head doesn't thrust forward.**
✓ **Place your hand under the steering wheel at four and eight o'clock and keep your elbows down.**
✓ **Move your seat close to allow your elbows to bend.**
✓ **If you have armrests, especially if they are on both side of your seat, use them!**
✓ **Don't lean off to one side. This can throw off your hips, causing lower back and hip pain.**
✓ **Lumbar support can really help your lower back, especially during long drives.**

Laptops and Counter Tops

High bar stool + Counter top = Lower back pain. We've done this one ourselves. Just a couple of minutes checking your email while sitting on your bar stool at your counter and your back will let you know it's not a good idea. Since you're high up and your laptop is down by your belly, this forces you to round your entire back severely so that you can see the screen. This improper posture is inviting a herniation or back spasm to come and ruin your day.

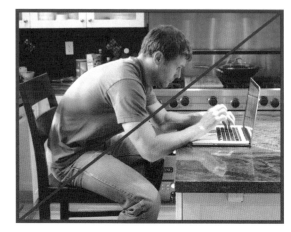

✓ **There isn't much to say, but don't do it, no matter how easy it may be. It's better to sit at the dinner table or anywhere else. Even if you sit up straight, you have to look down to see your screen, which will cause even more strain on your neck.**

Standing on One Leg

No, not like a flamingo. We mean leaning to one side, carrying the majority of your weight on one leg and, therefore, one hip. This stretches and strains the outer muscle of the hip and leg that you are standing on. This is a major cause of SI instability, lower back, hip, and groin pain.

The muscle tension and instability caused by this posture can lead to a condition known as **Patella Femoral Syndrome**, where your kneecap slides off to one side causing serious knee pain. Many people don't even realize that they shift their weight off to one side. More times than not, they tend to do it on the same leg which causes even further hip instability, leading to pain.

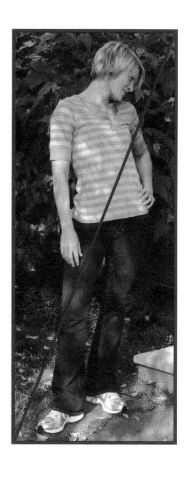

✓ **When you stand, stand firmly on both legs. If you *must* lean, equally switch which leg your weight is on.**
✓ **It would also be a great idea to do *The Office Effect* Lower Body Exercise Series to strengthen and balance all the muscles of your hip and lower back in order to keep you out of pain or pull you out of pain after a long day on your feet.**

Carrying a Purse or Backpack on One Shoulder

Even if your bag or purse is light, the upper shoulder and neck muscles will continually lift up to hold the strap on your shoulder, causing neck and shoulder pain.

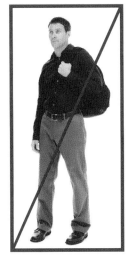 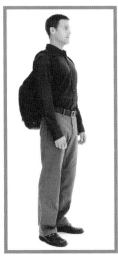 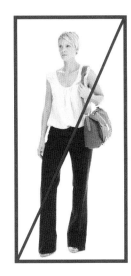 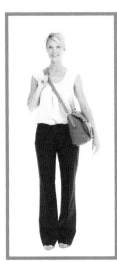

✓ **If it's a purse, put the strap across the body and switch sides periodically.**
✓ **If it's a backpack, use both straps.**
✓ **Y-T Pulldowns are a great exercise to counter purse or backpack shoulder stress.**

A Purse or Briefcase Can Change the Way You Walk.

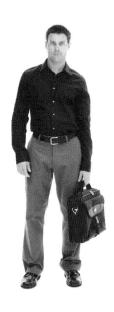

When you hold a bag, backpack, or briefcase on one side, especially if it's always the same side, you won't tend to swing that arm as you walk. Without this counterbalancing or pendulum like swing of the arm, your body will shorten the stride of one leg. This can change the way you walk and cause your hips to twist and your leg muscles to become unbalanced. Eventually this can give you lower back, hip, and groin pain.

✓ **Switch the side you hold your bag or suitcase on often.**

"You can empower yourself by making the decision to take control of your body and your environment. Use the tools we have given you and help yourself feel better, look better, and perform better."

Matt Williamson

Reference Materials

Publications:

Anatomical Chart Company, *The World's Best Anatomical Charts* (Skokie: Lippincott Williams & Wilkins, 2000).

Barham, Jerry N., and Edna P. Wooten, *Structural Kinesiology* (New York: The Macmillan Company, 1973).

Clark, Michael A., Scott C. Lucett, and Rodney J. Corn, *NASM Essentials of Personal Fitness Training*, 3rd ed. (New York: Lippincott Williams & Wilkins, 2007).

Delavier, Frederick, *Strength Training Anatomy* (Paris: Editions Vigot, 1998).

Fitt, Sally Sevey, *Dance Kinesiology* (New York: Schirmer Books, 1988).

Gallagher, Sean P., and Romana Kryzanowska, *The Pilates Method of Body Conditioning* (Philadelphia: BainBridgeBooks, 1999).

Kapit, Wynn, and Lawrence M. Elson, *The Anatomy Coloring Book*, 2nd ed. (New York: HarperCollins College Publishers, 1993).

Myers, Thomas, *Anatomy Trains Myofascial Meridians for Manual and Movement Therapists* (Edinburgh: Churchill Livingstone, 2004).

Netter, Frank H., *Atlas of Human Anatomy,* 3rd ed. (Teterboro: Icon Learning Systems, 2003).

Certifications:

- Stott International Certification Center for the Stott Pilates Method:
    - Mat Level 1 & Level 2 Certification
    - Reformer Level 1 & Level 2 Certification
    - Cadillac Level 1 & Level 2 Certification
    - Chair & Barrels Level 1 & Level 2 Certification
- National Academy of Sports Medicine Personal Training Certification
- National Academy of Sports Medicine Corrective Exercise Specialist Certification

The Office Effect^{TM} was developed by CMC Fitness Solutions^{TM}...

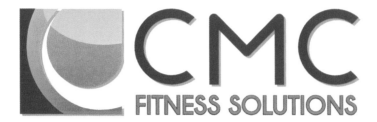

CMC Fitness Solutions is dedicated to helping people help themselves by offering simple, real world solutions to those who want to feel healthier and happier. We understand the demands of the working world and have developed our products with those demands in mind. Join us on the journey to a pain free day!

CMC's product line offers comprehensive systems that will make you *feel* better, *look* better and *perform* better, ranging from this book to corporate seminars, which can be incorporated into any corporate fitness, wellness, educational, or team-building programs you already have in place. Additionally, CMC will be offering upcoming DVDs and iPhone/iPad apps, as well as fitness and wellness products.

In the near future, CMC will be launching a certification system for other fitness professionals. Once certified, applicants will be able to fill the high demand for seminars in businesses around the nation, and be able to apply CMC's system to their own clients.

For more information about CMC Fitness Solutions, go to: www.cmcfitnesssolutions.com

OVERDUES
5¢ A DAY

12/11

ISLAND PARK PUBLIC LIBRARY
176 Long Beach Road
Island Park, NY 11558
Phone: 432-0122